ACCOUNT

OF THE

COAST DISEASES

OF

INDIA.

AN
ACCOUNT
OF THE
DISEASES OF INDIA

AN ACCOUNT OF THE DISEASES OF INDIA

AS THEY APPEARED

IN THE ENGLISH FLEET, AND IN THE NAVAL HOSPITAL AT MADRAS, IN 1782 AND 1783,

WITH

OBSERVATIONS ON ULCERS, AND THE HOSPITAL

SORES OF THAT COUNTRY, &C. &C.

CHARLES CURTIS

GYAN

Published by

GYAN

Gyan Publishing House
5, Ansari Road
Daryaganj, New Delhi-110002
Phone: 011-47034999, 9811692060
E-mail: books@gyanbooks.com

Distribution Network
gyanbooks.com
India, USA, Canada, UK, Australia

ISBN: 978-93-7097-206-3 (PB)

First Published, 1807

2nd Impression 2025

Printed at: Gyan Press, Delhi.

AN ACCOUNT OF THE DISEASES OF INDIA
Author CHARLES CURTIS,

AN

ACCOUNT

OF THE

DISEASES OF INDIA,

AS THEY APPEARED

IN THE ENGLISH FLEET, AND IN THE NAVAL HOSPITAL

AT MADRAS, IN 1782 AND 1783;

WITH

OBSERVATIONS ON ULCERS, AND THE HOSPITAL

SORES OF THAT COUNTRY, &c. &c.

TO WHICH IS PREFIXED,

A VIEW OF THE DISEASES ON AN EXPEDITION,

AND PASSAGE OF A FLEET AND ARMAMENT

TO INDIA, IN 1781.

BY

CHARLES CURTIS,

FORMERLY SURGEON OF THE MEDEA FRIGATE.

Edinburgh:

PRINTED FOR W. LAING;

AND LONGMAN, HURST, REES AND ORME,

AND J. MURRAY, LONDON.

1807.

TO

VICE-ADMIRAL

SIR ERASMUS GOWER,

&c. &c. &c.

AS a tribute of respect to his virtues, and in gratitude for many acts of kindness experienced under his command, in the Medea Frigate, this small Tract on the Diseases of India, is humbly and most respectfully dedicated, by

His most obedient

Humble Servant,

The Author.

EDINBURGH,
19th Jan. 1807.

TO

TO

Dr JAMES HAMILTON Primus,

Edinburgh.

SIR,

The benefit derived from your assistance, in many difficult cases of Medical Practice, and the instruction I have received in regard to the treatment of others, from your late publication On the Use of Purgative Medicines;—*in particular, with respect to* Chorea Sancti Viti,—*a well marked case of which came lately under my care, and has been perfectly cured by an adherence to the plan laid down in that excellent work;—renders it a duty, and seems also to confer a kind of right, to inscribe to you this short Treatise on the Diseases of India.*

It pretends to little more than to give a history of facts, with a few observations relating to foreign practice; of the accuracy or importance of which, those only who have had some medical experience in

 India

India can judge correctly. In taking the liberty, therefore, of presenting to you this Publication, it is obvious, I cannot have so much in view to procure for it your patronage, as to testify those sentiments of personal esteem with which I have the honour to be,

SIR,

Your most obedient Servant,

C. C.

EDINBURGH,
19th Jan. 1807.

CON-

CONTENTS.

Arrives

INDIA

INDIA DISEASES.

JAUNDICE,

APPENDIX.

CORRIGENDA.

Page 5. line 2. from the bottom, *for* at *read* with
17. 2. *for* inverſion *read* invaſion
31. 7. from the bottom, *add* Cort. Peruv.
46. 15. *for* fever-diſeaſes *read* liver-diſeaſes
83. 4. *for* eaſe *read* care
Appendix, No. IV. p. 172. l. 10. *add* certain

INTRODUCTION.

WHEN we conſider the great extent, and flouriſhing ſtate of the Britiſh poſſeſſions in India,—the ſplendid eſtabliſhments for the improvement of ſcience, and the ſucceſs with which many branches of it have been proſecuted there; and when we obſerve, that military and municipal hoſpitals; with able and ſkilful practitioners, have long been eſtabliſhed, and are to be met with in all the principal ſtations of the Company in that extenſive region, it may be a matter of ſome ſurpriſe to obſerve, that ſo little on the ſubject of MEDICINE, has been communicated from that quarter.—And that no good account has yet been given of the *morbid* conſtitution

ſtitution belonging to the country, or of the diſeaſes peculiar to it; ſo that ſtrangers, and the younger part of the profeſſion, often prematurely enough called to practiſe there, under very important truſts, might be enabled to undertake it with tolerable facility to themſelves, or with ſafety to thoſe under their care,—may well be matter of regret.

Placed in ſimilar circumſtances, it required no long time to make the author fully ſenſible of this want; and to convince him, That European noſology and definitions, would, in India, prove but uncertain or fallacious guides; that a ſtranger in ſhort, with a good deal to unlearn, would have his way at every ſtep to feel and trace out for himſelf. Nor is this perplexity, and the difficulties which we have to encounter, to be wondered at, on entering to practice in a country, where ſcarce a ſingle production, whether of the animal or vegetable kingdom, is to be met with, bearing a true reſemblance to its prototype in Europe; where, except for two or three weeks about the

the ſhifting of the monſoons, eſpecially of that which happens in the month of October, (I ſpeak of the Eaſtern Coaſt only), a ſhower of rain, or a breeze of wind, are almoſt unknown; where ſcarce ever a haze or cloud appears upon the horizon, to mitigate the dazzling ardour of an almoſt vertical ſun; and where the thermometer, through the whole 24 hours, ſeldom or never points under 80° of Fahrenheit, but generally far above it.

At no period of life is *diagnoſis* an eaſy part of the medical profeſſion. In the outſet it is always difficult. The author of the following ſheets had experienced this difficulty fully; and this had led to an early habit of taking caſes, or notes of ſuch diſeaſes as had fallen under his obſervation, adding ſuch reflections as were ſuggeſted to his mind, from ſymptoms and events as they occurred.

On being appointed, ſoon after his arrival in India, to do duty in the Naval Hoſpital at Madras, during the active ſervice of the fleet in the years 1782 and 1783, this practice was regularly continued: Not, however, to the extent of a full caſe-book and perfect tables, ſuch a taſk being two burdenſome for the laborious duty of this ſtation in ſuch a climate. Regular entries were made of the principal caſes only; and a general minute-book recorded the material circumſtances in ſuch as were of leſs importance. Full opportunity was enjoyed for diſſections, and many were accordingly performed, and the appearances recorded at the moment.

From ſuch materials, the following hiſtories of the principal and prevailing Coaſt Diſeaſes of India in thoſe years, are, with much diffidence, preſented to the public. Not that the author by any means preſumes they will be found an adequate ſupply for the want that has been noticed. Superior abilities, a longer reſidence in the country, a more full acquaintance with the nature of the climate,

mate, and its influence on the European conſtitution, than he enjoyed, would have been neceſſary for ſuch an undertaking. If what is here attempted, ſhall in any degree contribute to direct the inexperience of others, and preſerve them from falling into errors and miſtakes, which unavoidably occurred to the author in his own practice, by pointing out the illuſive and varying forms under which the ſymptoms of known diſeaſes preſent themſelves in this climate, ſome part of the difficulty at leaſt will be removed, and perſonal induſtry and experience will the ſooner ſupply what may ſtill be wanting. Let it be obſerved, however, that what is here ſtated, applies properly to *maritime* India only, and not to all the variety of inland country comprehended within that vaſt peninſula.

The claſſification and nomenclature of diſeaſes, is a neceſſary meaſure to facilitate the ſtudy of them; but we ought always to keep in view, that the beſt noſology is in ſome meaſure an artificial, often a fanciful arrangement, and behoves of neceſſity to be always more or leſs a local one. And hence, in relation to diſeaſes of foreign countries, there ariſes a danger of our being led into error, by the miſapplication of names, or by the inaccuracy of writers, in uſing theſe in a ſenſe different from that adopted by noſological and ſyſtematic authors.

To rectify what appears to me, to be an error of this kind, to be met with in more than one communication on the ſubject of India diſeaſes, is one object of the obſervations contained in the following ſheets.

Thus the name of *Dyſentery* has been uniformly made uſe of to diſtinguiſh an affection, which, from the accounts that are given of it, appears to be nothing different from that which takes place in the *bilious* and *hepatic fluxes* of India; both very generally attended, like dyſentery with ſome fever in the beginning, and ſeldom without a conſiderable degree of dyſenteric affection in ſome parts of their courſe;

courſe; but eaſily diſtinguiſhed from dyſentery, by the train of ſymptoms, by the nature of the evacuations, and by what has even been taken notice of, without leading to a correction of the error,—the circumſtance of their never being in any degree infectious. Were there nothing but a *name* concerned here, the matter might be conſidered as exceedingly trivial. But when we find mercurial frictions, puſhed the whole length of a ſalivating courſe, recommended by one, and doſes of calomel, to the extent of 10 grains every night, by another, as a ſafe and effectual mode of cure for what they term *dyſentery;* it is evident, if this practice were to be adopted in the treatment of *real* dyſentery, in many of its combinations, as with ſcorbutic diatheſis or typhus fever, much miſchief might undoubtedly follow;—and hence the importance of the diſtinction being made, becomes evident.

Of the ſpaſmodic diſeaſe known, when I was in India, under the name of *Mort de Chien*,

 no

no particular account has yet been given to the public. It is ſpoken of by BONTIUS, and has been mentioned by Mr GIRDLESTON; and it is more particularly referred to in a late academical theſis on the ſubject of *Tetanus*, of which it is conſidered as a ſpecies or variety*.

Tetanus, under what I have always underſtood to be its true and proper form, appeared on one occaſion at the hoſpital, and is taken notice of in ſome of the following communications. It was in every inſtance the conſequence of external injury, and preſerved throughout its courſe, a character ſo determinate, as to diſtinguiſh it completely from every other diſorder. It did not appear to me to have any agreement with the *mort de chien*, except in the ſingle circumſtance of external ſpaſm, and even in this there was a material difference. In tetanus, the ſpaſms are not attended with much pain in

* CONSIDEN *De Tetano*.

in the affected mufcl s, fcarcely indeed with any. It is far otherwife in the *mort de chien.* In tetanus, there is no contraction or gathering up of the belly of the mufcle into a hard knot, but rather a fixed rigidity, over-tone and tenfion of the whole mufcle, or of a number of the external mufcles at the fame time; efpecially of thofe that ferve to clofe the lower jaw, than what may be called a cramp or fpafm. Spafm was, in the cafe of tetanus, the great and principal fymptom of the difeafe, and its progrefs was regular and uniform. Whereas, in the *mort de chien*, it neither began nor finifhed the malady. It was moveable and variable in every degree, and the difcafc was accompanied all along, with fymptoms of far more ferious importance than even fpafm itfelf. In fine, fpafm appears in tetanus as the radical affection: In the other it is only fymptomatic.

Obftructed perfpiration, and the retention of acrimony fuppofed to be eliminated by the fkin, and the application of cold, efpecially when joined with hard exercise, and debilitating exertions, are supposed to furnish an easy explanation of many diseased phenomena, and have been adduced as the causes of tetanus, and of the disease under consideration. It may, however, be observed, that, on reviewing the provisions made by nature for correcting irregularities, or supplying the defects of this discharge, and the great inequalities to which it is daily and hourly subjected with impunity,—as in the practice of many nations inhabiting the hottest countries, in having their bodies constantly besmeared with oil or grease; we will find ourselves beset with difficulties in explaining diseases, by referring them to this source, in the same manner as we find these difficulties in most of our pathological inquiries.

Much will depend on idiosyncrasies and peculiarities of habit, which we cannot always understand or explain. Accordingly, I recollect to have observed several persons of a spare and thin habit of body, with dark hair

hair and ſwarthy complexions, who preſerved a degree of health and vigour in India quite inconſiſtent with the debilitating operation of the climate upon the generality of European conſtitutions; and theſe perſons ſuſtained the heat, without any ſenſible perſpiration at all: while others, again, enjoyed neither health nor ſpirits, nor vigour, but while under a continual vapour-bath of this exhalation. Whether the one or the other deſcription of perſons were moſt liable to the ſpaſmodic diſeaſes of the country, I made no obſervations to determine. Certain it is, that the lower claſſes of the natives, whoſe ſkins are very black, and who perſpire but little, are equally ſufferers by them as the Europeans, or perhaps more ſo.

Hepatitis, which occupies ſome room in the following work, has been ſo often treated of before, that little or nothing new can be added to the ſubject; unleſs it may be in what relates to diagnoſis,—or to the importance

portance of diſtinguiſhing between ſymptoms that are primary and characteriſtic, and thoſe that are only acceſſory or accidental; and the difficulty that frequently attends this diſtinction in India, from the general prominency and violence of the acceſſory ſymptoms there. On this ſubject, we have been ſomewhat particular, and have given ſeveral important and ſtriking examples.

On the ſubject of *Bilious Diſeaſes* and *Abdominal Affections*, ſo uncommonly prevalent in India, a very few preliminary obſervations may be perhaps introduced here without impropriety.

Redundancy and diſorder in the bilious ſecretion, is a diatheſis in ſome meaſure common to all tropical countries. But in India, I am diſpoſed to believe, that the conſtitutional temperament peculiar to the country extends to ſomething further; namely, ſanguineous plethora, with increaſed mobility and irritability over all that portion of the ſyſtem comprehended within the extent of the

the cœliacal and portal circle; and that from this ſource are derived redundancy of bile and acrimony of ſecretions, tendency to diſorder, diſeaſe, and derangement of functions over all this portion of the body, exceſſive fluxes, and the whole train of topical affections, to which the liver, inteſtines and meſentery are ſo conſtantly ſubjected in India. Hence diſeaſes that depend on a rigid or tenſe fibre, or any other determination of the circulating fluid; ſuch as rheumatiſm, catarrh and catarrhal affections; pleuritis or pneumonia, headachs or toothachs, are wholly unknown. Febrile diſeaſes are confined to exanthematous, ſymptomatical or hectic, and the nervous affections to the ſpaſmodic. Intermittents and remittents are, in Lower India, at leaſt, only ſymptomatics, ariſing from diſeaſed bile in the firſt paſſages. Renal or urinary affections we had none; and of all our numerous caſes of obſtruction of the liver or meſentery, and of cachexy from fluxes and impaired habit, not one ever end-

ed

ed in any ſpecies of dropſy. The ſtomach and inteſtines, the liver and meſentery, are here the grand ſources of almoſt every diſeaſe that occurs; or, what amounts nearly to the ſame thing, in every ſtanding complaint, if the radical affection does not lie in theſe organs, they are ſure to become the principal ſufferers in the iſſue.

At the time the obſervations on the *Ulcers* and *Hoſpital Sores* of India were made, I had ſeen no treatiſe on theſe ſubjects, or on hoſpital gangrene. Of courſe, the conjectures here ſtated concerning them may appear but crude and little ſatisfactory; and what has been viewed as peculiarities, reſulting from climate or ſituation, may be thought rather imputable to a general ſource of ſuch malignity, viz. foul and contaminated hoſpital air.

But whatever may be in this, I am perſuaded that thoſe we have ſtated were not without their influence, and that we were well founded in ſuppoſing the preſence of a greater degree

gree of acrimony in all ſecreted fluids, together with torpor, inactivity, and want of tone in the extreme veſſels, as unfavourable to the healing proceſs, in a degree far beyond what takes place in more temperate latitudes: And the facts on which we built this conjecture, were the following: That inſtead of a hard or full pulſe, with heat and roſe-coloured redneſs of parts, indicating an active inflammation, that ſoon terminates either in the eſtabliſhment of a good and plentiful ſuppuration, or in rapid and deſtructive gangrene; whenever external inflammation was any how induced, its characters were,—little heat or tumour of parts, inflammation of a palc or purpliſh hue, with a quick and feeble pulſe, indicating a feeble creeping kind of diſeaſe, terminating moſt commonly in an equally inactive ſort of gangrene, which it was yet extremely difficult to correct or reſiſt; and this was often the reſult from wounds, fractures and contuſions received in action, as well as in eſtabliſhed ſores; and

was

was obſervable in ſhips, whether they had been a long or ſhort time at ſea, as well as at the hoſpital. True phlegmon, or any thing of the nature of eryſipelas, we never ſaw. This laſt is indeed a frequent hoſpital diſeaſe, and ſome people have aſſigned to it a bilious origin; but it never appeared with us.

Expeditions, ſo tedious as that under the command of Commodore JOHNSTON, can but ſeldom happen. Paſſages to India are ſeldom extended to the length of eleven months; but they are ſometimes ſufficiently protracted, to give riſe to a variety of ſhip-complaints. An account of the kinds and ſucceſſion of diſeaſes, likely to be met with in ſimilar circumſtances, it is conceived, may be of ſome uſe to thoſe who have not been accuſtomed to ſuch kind of ſervice.

Sea-ſcurvy, which was formerly the bane and ſcourge of many a hopeful undertaking, is now, from the reforms in ſea-victualling, a much leſs frequent occurrence than formerly.

merly. Slighter degrees of it, not very easily detected, unless by some acquaintance with the disease under its proper form, and which never fail to give a covered and latent malignity to many other disorders, will, however, now and then occur. The short account of it here given will serve in some measure to detect these, and may perhaps supersede the necessity of consulting older, more minute, and tedious descriptions.

Two letters, published in this Collection, may seem to require some explanation, and perhaps an apology. The longest and most important of them has already been communicated to the public by Dr CARMICHAEL SMYTH in Dr DUNCAN's *Annals of Medicine* for the year 1801. This, it may be thought, ought to have superseded the necessity of a republication. But the subject, and the sentiments contained in it, do so much elucidate and confirm the doctrines here delivered, as to render it a very important and necessary addition. Copies of both letters were in the

hands

hands of moſt of the older ſurgeons of the fleet under Sir EDWARD HUGHES; and they were deſervedly valued, as containing by far the beſt general information on the India diſeaſes, to be procured in the country. Although they were but private letters, the hand of a maſter is viſible in both. The author has printed from the copy of them, which has been in his private poſſeſſion for above twenty years. The letter which relates to the *Cholera Morbus* or *Mort de Chien* *, as

* It is printed *Maux de Chiens*, in Dr SMYTH's copy of the other letter. In India, I know, dogs are ſubject to the liver-diſeaſe, but never that I heard of to any thing like the cholera morbus or cramp. The name does not ſtand in my copy of the ſecond letter at all; but the *mort de chien* is undoubtedly the diſeaſe pointed at in the place where Dr SMYTH's copy has *maux de chiens*. *Mort de chien* was the name in the fleet; and it may have been of ſhip-coinage originally, importing the pitiful manner in which a brave and boiſterous ſeaman was condemned to loſe his life;—to die like a dog!

as appears from the ſtyle and manner, has been written in much haſte; yet ſtill it contains ſo much information on the ſubject, and points out ſuch diſtinctions, in relation to caſes and ſymptoms, as to ſhew of how great value a more finiſhed account from the ſame hand would have been.

In this publication, the author has not thought it of much conſequence to be very particular in ſtating forms of preſcriptions, and doſes of medicines,—as being in a great meaſure unneceſſary to the claſs of readers for whom it is intended. Nor is there in fact much variety or elegance of preſcription, to be expected in a detail of foreign hoſpital practice. Every thing in ſuch a ſituation comes neceſſarily under ſome general plan and ſyſtem of management; and no where is this attended with leſs inconvenience than in India, where diſeaſes are at bottom ſo ſimple, and ſo little varied in their eſſential characters, that a ſhort experience enables a practitioner to

treat

treat a number, that would be thought in any other country quite incompatible with any ſort of due attention or care.

To exhibit uſeful facts, and to ſtate only ſuch as came under the author's own obſervation, without indulging in theoretic diſquiſition, or laboured ſpeculations, has been his object throughout.

By examining memoirs, reports, and accounts in periodical works, he could have ſwelled this ſmall volume to a more reſpectable ſize; but this, except in ſo far as appeared neceſſary to the rectification of what was deemed erroneous, has been purpoſely avoided.

All the diſeaſes here treated of, came under the author's own care; not in ſingle or ſolitary caſes, but in claſſes and whole wards together; and they include all the diſeaſes of any conſequence that were met with in the country. Errors and miſtakes in the treatment of them he was often ſenſible of himſelf;

himſelf; but he has made no attempts to palliate or conceal any of them. Thoſe who have had ſome experience of the difficulties which frequently occur in the profeſſion, will know how to make reaſonable allowances.

He has much to fear, ſhould the reader be inclined to exerciſe the ſeverity of criticiſm with reſpect to imperfections and defects in point of compoſition to be found in this publication. Accuſtomed to commit his thoughts to writing for his own peruſal only, the author is ſenſible he may have contracted an abreviated form of diction, leſs ſuited than he could wiſh to a public appearance; and a deſire of adhering cloſely to the ſtatements in his original notes, may doubtleſs have infuſed too much of the journal ſtyle into his work. But in all other reſpects, he is deſirous rather to ſolicit correction, than to deprecate or ſhun it.

MEDICAL OBSERVATIONS

ON AN

EXPEDITION AND PASSAGE

TO

INDIA, &c.

13th March 1781.

ON this day, a fleet, under the command of Commodore Johnſtone, ſailed from St Helen's, conſiſting of the following ſhips, Hero, 74; Monmouth, 64; Iſis, 50; Romney, 50; Jupiter, 50; Jaſon, Active, Mercury, and Diana frigates; Rattleſnake and Lark cutters; Terror bomb, and Infernal fireſhip; with five King's tranſports, ſeveral ſtoreſhips and victuallers; having under convoy a fleet for the Weſt Indies and thirteen Eaſt Indiamen. On board the

 tranſports,

tranſports, ſtoreſhips, and in the Eaſt Indiamen, were embarked the 98th, 100th, and the 2d battalion of the 42d regiments, with four independent companies of additionals.

In the King's tranſport ſhip the Manilla, were embarked the hoſpital ſtaff and ſtores, with two companies from the 98th and 100th, hoſpital ſurgeon, and two mates, under whoſe care the troops were. The ſhip's complement, conſiſting of the Lieutenant commander, maſter, warrant-officers, and forty ſeamen, being all the people whoſe health I had in charge.

From the ſhip being put in commiſſion to our ſailing from St Helen's, no diſeaſe had appeared among the ſeamen, excepting one caſe of ſynochus fever. The pulſe, from the firſt, was frequent and feeble, with pain of the head and back. The antimonial ſolution * *ad vomitum*, was given him in the beginning; but by his taking it, through miſtake, in too large doſes, it brought on continued vomitings and singultus. After trying different anti-emetics and antiſpaſmodics, without effect, theſe were completely removed by a large bliſter *inter ſcapulas*, which raiſed his pulſe, and relieved

* Solutio Tartritis Antimonii.

lieved the anxiety and oppreſſion of breaſt he had complained much of for ſome days before. After this, his recovery was eaſy and rapid, with the aſſiſtance of wine and cordials only. When we left St Helen's, the ſhip's company were all in perfect health, and there were few or no complaints among the troops; but they were new raiſed, and poor looking men; many of them mere boys, and a number much over the proper age for ſervice in hot climates: ſeveral only in a ſtate of convaleſcence from fevers, which had infeſted them much in Hilſea-barracks, where they had been quartered.

On the 10th April, the whole fleet anchored in Port Prayo Bay, in the Iſland of St Jago, lat. 15° 30′ N.

The weather, from our leaving England, down Channel, and acroſs the Bay of Biſcay, was clear and moderate for the ſeaſon; with light winds and calms in the Bay. By the 25th of March, the increaſe of heat and change of climate had become perceptible. When we reached this iſland, the heat, from a nearly vertical ſun, was exceſſive; yet the evenings and mornings were cool.

For nearly the laſt fortnight, we had found a ſteady wind at N. E.; the air dry and clear, without night-dews or damps. Among the ſeamen, we had only a few ſlight rheumatic complaints down Channel; and two or three febrile diſorders in the latter part of the paſſage. One of them, however, turned out continued and fatal. The patient complained, in the beginning, of much pain in the head, great lowneſs and depreſſion of ſpirits, with a quick ſmall pulſe. His ſkin ſoon became dry, and his tongue parched. Belly natural, but he had much thirſt, and all along an unpromiſing caſt of countenance. An antimonial emetic and neutral mixtures, with bliſtering, procured no relief. A doſe of opium and camphor, on the 10th day, brought out a moiſture on his ſkin and tongue, which promiſed to be of ſervice; but in the end afforded none. The ſweating became profuſe and cold, and he died on the 12th. Our ſeamen ſlept at this period in the fore hold, under the platform for the troops, which was exceedingly ill-aired and hot; and I had no doubt added to the malignity of this man's diſeaſe. Two ſoldiers alſo died of ſimilar fevers during the paſſage.

The

The event of this case, and the increase of sickness among the troops, rendered it extremely necessary to provide a better sick-birth for the accommodation of the seamen; and every part of the deck below being taken up by the soldiers' platforms, foreseeing a sickly passage, I took the first occasion to pre-occupy for this purpose the stern-sheets of a flat-bottomed boat, carried on the ship's deck under the booms. An awning being spread over these, covered in the whole, and served our purpose most excellently; while the fore part of the boat, also covered by the awning, but left open at the sides, afforded a sheltered sleeping-place for the rest of the sailors. Of this station, they kept possession through the whole voyage; even during the cold weather we experienced in doubling the Cape, so far south as 42°, and was without doubt a principal means of preserving them from the influence of contagion often raging among the troops below; or at least rendered the effects of it much less fatal than otherwise it might have been.

May 1.—Lat. 9° N. At sea, stearing south at a steady light breeze at N. E.; weather exceedingly hot, but the atmofphere dry and clear. No complaints occurred among the feamen at St Jago; and the troops got free from the fevers which had affected them on the paffage to the ifland. The fatigue of watering there was great, and expofure to the heat of the fun conftant; the water being to roll in cafks a confiderable way to the beach, and to raft off through a heavy furf and fwell above a mile and a half to the fhips. The people in general flept expofed to the night-air both on fhore and on board, yet no injury to health was fuftained. Frefh meat, vegetables, and the tropical fruits were procured in great plenty, efpecially where old clothes could be given in barter for them; and the water was good, though fomewhat brackifh at the neareft well.

While at anchor in the bay, the fleet were attacked by a French fquadron, commanded by Monfeur Souffrain. None were killed or wounded on board the Manilla; but fome days after the action, fourteen foldiers wounded by mufket-fhot, were put on board, under the care of the hofpital-ftaff. They were moftly flefh wounds, chiefly through the limbs; only two had the bones fractured. They all healed eafily; nor was there in any of them

them a neceſſity for counter openings, except in one caſe, for the extraction of a button or piece of cloth. I did not obſerve, either in theſe, or in ſome caſes I ſaw on board other ſhips the day after the action, ſo much blackening and ſcaring as ball-wounds are in general ſaid to exhibit; but I obſerved in all the caſes, that the ball had made a much larger opening on the ſide by which it paſſed out than that by which it entered. Fomentation and poultices, or embrocation with ſaturnine ſolution, light rolling and dreſſings, with occaſional laxatives, and an opiate every night, till the ſuppuratory proceſs was completely eſtabliſhed, and after that wine and bark, were the only means of cure employed, and in all with full ſucceſs.

June 1.—Lat. 12° 15′ South.

Before the end of laſt month, fevers had begun again to prevail in many of the tranſport and troop ſhips. In the Manilla, out of about 180 ſoldiers, 56 are now in the ſick-liſt, under fever of conſiderable variety of form; and two have died of it ſince leaving St Jago. Some way before we reached the Line, we were deſerted by the N. E. trade-wind; and near it, were frequently becalmed for two or three days together; with now and then hurricane ſqualls, tornadoes, and guſts of wind; with occaſional loud thunder, and heavy falls of rain.

The troops now begin to have a pale, ſqualid and ſickly appearance. The fever begins with pain in the head and back; ſome have alſo pains in the limbs; and in others, it is attended with diarrhœa. Generally the tongue is yellow, and the urine high coloured; but without bilious vomitings or yellowneſs of the ſkin. The army ſurgeons conſider this as an ardent, rather than a bilious fever, and ſay, that bark has been generally ſucceſsful in removing it. Towards the end of the month, the genus of the fever became much better diſtinguiſhed, and, in moſt of the troop-ſhips, took on the dyſenteric form,—ſevere diarrhœa, gripes, teneſmus, with mucous and bloody ſtools. We have now, among the ſeamen, fluxes, with a ſlight evening fever, but with the dyſenteric affection very mild. They complain more of pains in their limbs, owing to their ſleeping in a cooler ſituation. One or two of them have, however, complained of ſome teneſmus; but none have had as yet mucous or bloody ſtools. All of theſe have yielded eaſily to to ſmall doſes of neutral purgative ſalts, with gentle diaphoretics.

July 1.—Lat. 29° 13 South. Weather rather cold, with frequent ſqualls and rain.

Dyſenteric fluxes are now, in a manner, common throughout the whole fleet; and rage, eſpecially in the troop-ſhips. The fever among the ſoldiers in this ſhip, is of a very malignant kind; and the diſeaſe has proved fatal to great numbers through the fleet in general.

Scurvy now alſo begins to make its appearance; attacking thoſe firſt who have been reduced by previous fevers or flux. In ſuch caſes, the patient goes off in a ſort of general cachexy, rather than with the ſymptoms of true formed ſcurvy. They continue pale and ſallow, with very little appetite; a low latent ſtate of fever remains, and they never recover any ſtrength, but complain much of torpor and weakneſs, with difficult or oppreſſed breathing. The fleſh waſtes away, and they go off under a ſlow maraſmus, without the external ſymptoms of ſcurvy being very remarkable. When this diſeaſe began to ſhew itſelf in thoſe who had been previouſly healthy, and of a ſound

ſound conſtitution, the firſt appearances of it were, a ſtiffneſs, with ſome ſwelling about the ſides of both the ankle and knee joints, affecting the tendons chiefly. By degrees the ſwelling increaſes, and pits a little, but never becomes very conſiderable. The parts around the joints become diſcoloured,—of a duſky yellow, then livid, at laſt black; with extenſive yellow ſuffuſions under the ſkin, along the back-part of the leg and thigh; but affecting much more the tendinous parts about the joints, than the ſoft and muſcular parts, or the middle of the member, running along and ſpreading in exanthematous patches, ſtreaks and blotches, each with a yellow margin extending far around it. Soon after theſe begin to appear, the gums ſwell, become ſpongy and livid, and bleed eaſily. The whole ſkin, but eſpecially the face and eyes, becomes dun and yellowiſh. A great degree of liſtleſſneſs and of languor ſupervenes; though they have a tolerable appetite, are at times cheerful when not preſſed to action, and have a flow of ſpirits.

Wherever this diatheſis prevails to any conſiderable degree, the ſlighteſt ſore or ulcer ſoon puts on a particular appearance; the edges become tumid,

mid, livid, or black and retracted. This colour diffufes itfelf fome way round the fore, declining to a dun yellow of much larger extent. A fpongy flefh, of a fibrous confiftence, refembling cruor or gore, fprings up in the middle of the fore, preventing all difcharge, except perhaps of a little fanies, which often iffues from it. Sometimes it dries and hardens with the air, fo as to afford no difcharge whatever; and in this ftate the fore continues without any change till the habit is corrected; for fuch fores never run into fpreading gangrene. Where there are no open fores or ulcers, there often appear a number of lumps on the fkin, owing to the effufion of blood, efpecially where any bruife or hurt has been received; yet, when opened, thefe emit nothing, but confift of a hard coagulum, like that which takes place on the open fores. Neither fometimes do the exanthematous blotches about the joints, bleed upon being opened with a lancet, and the whole parts become hard, dry and contracted, rather than fwelled.

Where fever or flux had preceded and exhaufted the habit, the external fcorbutic appearances were in a much inferior degree; but the fymp-

toms

toms of internal oppreſſion and putreſcency of the fluids were more remarkable. The gums became early more ſwelled and ſpongy, and bled more. The breath became fœtid, and ſtank; and every thing about them had a cadaverous ſmell. Reſpiration became difficult and laborious; extreme weakneſs and fainting fits came on; and in one or other of theſe fainting fits it was that all our ſcorbutics who died were carried off. Our ſeamen in the Manilla have as yet exhibited no appearances of ſcurvy, though ſome ſeamen in the larger ſhips are beginning to be tainted; but numbers of the troops are daily falling down with it; and it has already proved fatal to many.

Our moſt ſevere and fatal diſeaſe in the Manilla, continues to be the fever and flux, with the ſymptoms exceedingly ſevere, and marking a high degree of malignity. The diſeaſe is ſtrongly infectious. Where it aroſe, does not well appear; but an epidemic dyſentery now rages through the whole fleet, though in very different degrees in different ſhips. Almoſt the whole of our ſeamen have had more or leſs of it; but the degree and malignity of the diſeaſe, and eſpecially of the febrile affection, has with them been greatly milder

than

than among the troops; owing, I presume, to their sleeping in a freer and purer air than any other description of persons in the ship. The greater part of those seized lately, have had some fever during the first stage. Some of them with griping and tenesmus, mucous and bloody stools of considerable extent and continuance. Of those first attacked, the recoveries were easy; and little beyond some regulation of their diet, a purge or two of some mild neutral salt, with gentle diaphoretics occasionally; such as Pulv. Jacob. gr. x. *, night and morning; or if there was any degree of griping or tenesmus, after giving one saline purgative, a pill composed of Pulv. Ipecacuan. gr. i., and two or three of Rhubarb twice or thrice a-day, with a bolus at bed-time, composed of ten grains of Pulvis e Scordio cum Opio, *Ph. Lond.*, and a few grains of James's Powder, answered exceedingly well. But when the disease became more severe, and came on with more fever in the beginning, I began by giving them an emetic of Ipecacuan., and for some days following, Pulv. Ipecac. gr. i.; Pulv. Rhei et Pulv. Jacob. a gr. v. terties

* Pulv. Antimon. cum Phosph. Calc. *Ph. Edin.* Pulv. Antimon. *Lond.* Pulv. Stibiat. *Dub.*

terties indies. When griping became ſevere, a doſe of Sal Glauberi *, with an opiate at bed-time, generally gave much relief. I made it, however, a rule, to give no opiate till two or three purgatives had been firſt premiſed, and then only to relieve teneſmus, and procure eaſe through the night; never when there was conſiderable griping; unleſs ſeveral free ſtools had been procured through the day: whenever this was ſevere, a laxative was always given an hour or two before the exhibition of the opiate.

The practice with the troops in the ſhip conſiſted more in an alternation of laxatives and aſtringents, or opiates,—ſalts every day or every other day, and an opiate, or a doſe of Confectio Japonica † at bed-time. But among them the ſeverity of the diſeaſe, and malignity of the fever attending it, was much greater than among the ſeamen. With the latter, the fever generally came to a termination by the time the bowel-diſorder was removed; ſometimes ſooner. It was very different among the ſoldiers; with them, both generally ran on to a great length. The recoveries

* Sulphas Sodæ. † Elect. Catechu.

veries were much leſs perfect; and though the dyſenteric ſymptoms might be abated, a waſting flux and low hectic fever remained; or they fell into a ſcorbutic ſtate, from which they never could be recovered while the fleet remained at ſea.

With the ſeamen, I thought much benefit was derived from paying ſtrict attention to their diet. Taking away their ſhips' proviſion entirely, and feeding them on rice-gruel, with portable ſoup diſſolved in it, and ſago, with Port wine. After the ſeverity of gripes and teneſmus had been pretty much abated, I gave them twice a-day a large bolus of Conſerv. Roſarum *, with fifteen or ſixteen drops of Elixir of Vitriol mixed up with it, and found it grateful, and uſeful as an aſtringent, and for recovering the tone of the ſtomach and bowels.

In the courſe of laſt and this month, we have buried fifteen ſoldiers from dyſenteric fever and flux, or cachectics from theſe combined with ſcurvy. The exceſſive heats, the length of time ſpent near the Line, from calms, and light or baffling winds, has undoubtedly contributed much to ſo great a ſickneſs through the whole fleet.

July

* Conſerv. Roſæ, *Dub.*

July 20.—Fleet at anchor in Saldanha Bay. Lat. 30° 14′ South.

The weather has now become rather cold, hazy and cloudy, with frequent rains. Intelligence being obtained from the papers of a Dutch veſſel taken on the paſſage, that five ſail of their Eaſt India ſhips, with ſome ſmall craft were lying in this bay, covered from all view from the coaſt by a ridge of high land, the Commodore entered it on this day, and made prize of the whole, except one ſhip ſet on fire and blown up by the Dutch ſailors, before ſhe could be reached by the boats of the fleet.

Fluxes continue with increaſed malignity and fatality, in almoſt all the troop-ſhips. Several of the officers and ſurgeons have alſo caught the infection, though it has not yet proved fatal to any of them. None have proved obſtinate among our ſeamen, except in one inſtance, wherein relapſes have been frequent; nor has his medicines procured him much relief, till of late that ſome benefit has been obtained, from ſmall doſes of James's Powders through the day, in a large draught of ſaline mixture, with an opiate at bed-time. His habit is thin, and his conſtitution puny. His look gets ſallow, and he has become feeble and emaciated;

emaciated; with dry ſkin, thirſt, and a quick and feeble pulſe. Moſt probably from the inverſion of ſcorbutic diatheſis, though there are no external ſymptoms of that diſeaſe as yet.

Auguſt 20.—Lat. 42° South. Rounding the Cape of Good Hope at all this diſtance. Wind variable, and frequent gales. The weather cold and wet, with ſleet and ſnow ſhowers.

The object of the expedition was now known to us to have been an attack upon the Cape; but intelligence was procured at Saldanha Bay, that Monſieur Souffrain with his crippled fleet which had attacked us at Port Prayo, had arrived there long before us. Commodore Johnſtone detached the expedition, with the Indiamen, tranſports and men of war, for India; returning himſelf to St Helena, with the prize ſhips, the Romney and moſt of the frigates. The India diviſion made ſail through the inner paſſage, between Madagaſcar and the Main, for the Iſland of Johanna, where it was intended we ſhould refreſh and water. Since our advance to colder latitudes, the frequency of fluxes has diminiſhed, and many who had laboured long under them have began to recover. But thoſe who have had frequent relapſes, or previous fevers, do not return to a ſtate of health. They continue to have a pale and ſallow look, and do not acquire ſtrength or fleſh. The diſeaſe degenerates into a colliquative diarrhœa, without gripes; and they complain of oppreſſion about the breaſt, with extreme weakneſs; the ſure ſymptoms of the acceſſion of ſea-ſcurvy in ſuch exhauſted habits, and which ſoon proves fatal to ſuch ſubjects.

In ſome of the ſhips, fevers of the bilious and remittent kind have been very prevalent, and many have been cut off by them.

Scurvy advances with a rapid courſe, without our having it, in our power, either to check its progreſs, or give much relief to thoſe labouring under it. Neither medical preſcription, nor the ſcanty allowance of ſick proviſions hitherto provided to the navy ſurgeons, have been found of much avail againſt this diſeaſe. Freſh meat, the ſtock of vegetables and fruit laid in at St Jago, have been long exhauſted; and moſt of the ſhips have long ſince expended their ſtock of Engliſh beer; nor do I underſtand that eſſence of ſpruce, or of malt, have done much, even in thoſe ſhips which

which had the greateſt ſtore of theſe articles to iſſue out. But it is worthy of remark, that in ſome of the India ſhips, alſo carrying troops, where theſe were ſerved out early, ſo ſoon as the ſhip's beer was all expended, ſcurvy has been later in making its appearance, and has not made ſo much progreſs as in other ſhips, even where theſe were ſerved in the greateſt plenty, after it had begun to ſhew itſelf. So that it would appear much eaſier to guard againſt the acceſſion of this diſorder, by ſuch diet and drinks as lay in a proviſion againſt the ſeptic proceſs in the habit, than to counteract and reſiſt its progreſs, after it has once begun.

In nearly four months after leaving St Jago, the fleet reached the Iſland of Johanna, Lat. 15° South.

In this tedious voyage, no ſupplies of freſh meat, vegetables, or even of freſh water, were obtained, except indeed of tea, which the wreck of one of the prize-ſhips in Saldanha Bay afforded to the whole fleet in great plenty. But ſugar was become a ſcarce article even among the officers, and the men had none. Its place was, however, ſupplied with molaſſes, and contributed ſomewhat, no doubt, to refift the fcorbutic diathefis. Neither feamen nor foldiers ate the four-crout in fufficient quantities to do much good, though plenty of it was ferved out to them; and the fcorbutics, from the condition of their mouth and gums, could not, unlefs when boiled, which fpoils it much. A draught of water, with elixir of vitriol, or vinegar and water, three or four times a-day, after wafhing the gums with a part of it, was all we could do for them in the way of medical affiftance.

The cold weather in paffing the Cape, rather changed our dyfenteric fluxes into chronic diarrhœa than removed the difeafe; and this becoming combined with fcorbutic weaknefs, proved very generally fatal. Before reaching this ifland, many even of the petty-officers, who had been reduced to the fame provifions with the common feamen, began to exhibit the fymptoms and external appearances of fcurvy; but this was only in a mild and flight degree.

Baffling winds, calms and currents, kept the fleet for feveral days from reaching the anchoring-ground, with the ifland conftantly in view; and during thefe melancholy days, the fhips were every now and then committing to the deep fome unfortunate

fortunate ſcorbutic, whom a few cocoa-nuts and the tropical fruits, which were there in great plenty, might have preſerved to reach the much wiſhed for ſhore.

The green and pictureſque appearance of this iſland affords a proſpect peculiarly intereſting to every ſhip's company who have been any length of time at ſea. To us, (at leaſt to all our ſcorbutics), it preſented ſomething more. To them it was like the hope of a reſurrection from the dead: and in fact, one-third of all the troops and ſhips'-companies, were tranſported to its ſhores in a condition, in which a jolt, or a rude motion, was in danger almoſt to prevent their ever reaching them; and above another third more than half way to the ſame condition.

This, like moſt of the tropical iſles, is compoſed of high land, running towards the centre in irregular ridges: The hills, covered to the top with the green and ſpreading cocoa-nut tree: Some level land upon the ſhores, and deep and narrow valleys running backwards with more or leſs aſcent among the hills. On the north ſide, where the fleet anchored, a border of low land, in ſome places of half a mile or more in breadth, forms the beach;

 while

while three fresh-water streams, of considerable size, furnish easy and plentiful supplies of that article for any fleet. Farther back the land begins to rise in irregular elevations, and the valleys, which are wide and open to the beach, narrow and contract as they recede from it, and soon begin to be covered with shrubs, bushes and underwood. The cocoa-tree seems to thrive alike at all the heights in the island, from the top of the highest hills to within a few yards of the beach. On the banks of the middle rivulet, among the cocoa-tree groves, but where there is a firm and dry sward, and on the open beach near it, the greatest number of the ships pitched their sick tents, while some of the troops, the 98th and 42d regiments, went farther back into the opening of the valley, and towards the rising grounds, farther off from the reach of the sea-breeze, where there were fewer trees, but more bushes and underwood. Frequent rains, which fell out before we left the place, rendered their situation still more unfavourable, from the ground being more imperfectly dried, while near the shore, or among the cocoa groves, there was much more ventilation, and a much better shade from the excessive heats. From the last report, on the

the 20th Auguſt, to our reaching this place, the deaths at ſea were ten ſoldiers and one ſeaman.—The laſt was the caſe mentioned in the former report, as not recovering from dyſentery. Symptoms of ſcurvy, or rather of ſcorbutic diatheſis, became more and more apparent, and the patient went off in a low oppreſſed waſted ſtate ſome days before we reached this. All the ſoldiers, except one, (who died from drinking ſpirits to exceſs), were affected with ſcurvy, combined with cachexy, and died in the ſame way.

A very few days on ſhore made a remarkable change on the condition of our people. Tropical fruits, pot-herbs, and freſh beef, were procured in great plenty, and the cocoa-nut was in ſuch abundance, that both officers and men diluted their ſpirits with no other liquor; and at a certain period of its growth, it yields a clear ſubacid ſweet juice, which, with a due proportion of ſpirits, is made into excellent punch at once. On ſuch diet and drinks, recoveries from the ſevereſt degrees of ſcurvy were rapid. The ſpongy gums, black vibices and exanthematous blotches, very ſoon began to diſappear: The colour firſt changing from purple or black, to a dirty yellow, and this alſo vaniſhing altogether in a very ſhort time longer; ſo that it was very common to ſee men, who had been carried on ſhore in their hammocks, walking about with crutches, or the help of a ſingle ſtick, in three or four days. Some ſtiffneſs and a degree of ſwelling, however, remained about the joints for a longer period.

Some of the ſeamen had a fancy of ſitting with their legs buried in a hole dug in the earth, for an hour or two at a time: I did not perceive with any effect. In fact, freſh vegetable proviſions in ſufficient plenty were perfectly effectual; nor did it ſeem to make any difference at all of what kind theſe were, provided they were in ſufficient quantity *.

No

* The nature and cauſes of Sea-ſcurvy are now ſo well underſtood, that it would be entirely ſuperfluous to offer any explanation on the ſubject. But the following ſhore caſe of it, if an Iriciſm may be allowed, goes ſo directly to point out the nature and proximate cauſe, that it may be worth while, for the uſe of ſuch as have few opportunities of ſeeing the complaint, to put it down.

J. P. an inhabitant of Edinburgh, complained to me, ſome time in the winter of 1795, of pain and ſtiffneſs of his ankle joints. I did not look at the condition of the parts, but gave him ſome Liniment. Saponaceum * to rub on them. In four or five days he called again, to ſay his complaint was increaſing, and affected the knee-joint alſo. He had mentioned no diſcolouring,

* Liniment. Saponis, *Ph. Edin.*

No new diſeaſes aroſe among our people at the iſland, except trifling fluxes, from a too liberal uſe of vegetables, and drinking too freely of the cocoa-nut liquor, which is readily fermentable. But a fever, ſaid to be of the bilious remitting kind,

---

louring, and I was a good deal ſurpriſed, on inſpection, to ſee on both legs the diſtinct and well-marked appearance of ſea-ſcurvy, ſuch as it has been deſcribed. On deſiring him to ſhew me his gums, they were ſpongy, ſwelled, and full of purple mulberry-like lumps, from which blood iſſued. He ſaid alſo he was weak and breathleſs, and could not ſupport his uſual exertions. On inquiring into his diet, and way of life, I learned that he was a remarkable dyſpeptic, and could not uſe a ſingle article of vegetable food except tea and bread, nor make uſe of any malt liquor, and drank only ſpirits and water after his meals; that his employment was in a rag warehouſe, picking and ſorting woollen rags for navy beds, and that he ſlept in a room immediately over his warehouſe. From this account the nature of his complaint became very evident, even though the appearances had been leſs deciſive. Notwithſtanding his averſion to vegetables, and his account that every thing of that ſort gave him ſtomach complaints, he was directed to eat as many oranges, either bitter or ſweet, in the day, as he ſhould find upon trial his ſtomach would bear, and alſo to try the uſual articles of vegetable diet, and porter for drink. This ſort of food he now found to agree with him perfectly well; and what is remarkable, his dyſpeptic diſorder was removed by it, as well as the ſcurvy. He has become luſty and full, and enjoys very good health, though he continued his employment in the rag warehouſe for two or three years afterwards, only changing his place of ſleeping for one much better aired and healthy.

kind, had appeared among the troops of the 98th and 42d, ſtationed in the mouth of the valley, and ſome had died of it before our embarkation.

After remaining about three weeks on ſhore, the whole expedition was again ſhipped and prepared for ſea, with a plentiful ſtore of every edible vegetable the iſland afforded, pumpkins and cocoa nuts, which keep for any length of time, and as many live bullocks as every ſhip could find room to ſtow on their decks. With ſuch proviſion for the voyage to India, we flattered ourſelves with a healthy and proſperous paſſage. But in this we were diſappointed. The fever which ſome of the troops had caught on the iſland, was carried with them on board, and continued to ſpread, and proved fatal to many.

CASES OF REMITTENT FEVER.

Two days before our embarkation, the commander of the Manilla, Lieutenant R——, who had lived on ſhore very intemperately, continually rambling about through the whole encampment; often

often in a ſtate of intoxication, and frequently lying down to ſleep in the open air, had caught the ſame kind of fever which prevailed in the valley among the 98th regiment.

The attack began with pain of his head, with exceſſive heat of the ſkin, and alſo in the internal parts; quick and ſmall pulſe; nauſea and ſickneſs at ſtomach. On his firſt complaint, or as ſoon as it could be diſtinguiſhed from the effects of debauch, he was vomited with repeated ſmall doſes of tartar emetic ſolution. This alſo operated as a cathartic, and diſcharged much bilious ſtuff. This was in the afternoon, and relieved all his complaints; and next morning he thought himſelf perfectly well. The remiſſion, however, was but ſhort; and, during it, he repeated the ſame ſort of exceſſes that had brought on the diſeaſe. The fever returned after dinner, but remitted again in the evening. The bilious purging continued, but not ſevere. On the following morning, he complained again as before; but there was a conſiderable remiſſion, and he walked out freely, though his tongue was white, and his pulſe too quick. This day he had ſome ſmall doſes of rhubarb and ipecacuanha to promote his ſtools. He had from the

the firſt refuſed to take bark, which was ſtrongly preſſed upon him; and in the evening he went on board the ſhip. He had a reſtleſs night, moaned much in his ſleep; and next morning, the fourth of his illneſs, all the ſymptoms were worſe. He had a wild delirious look, and was not diſtinct in his anſwers. Pulſe very quick and catching; looſeneſs gone; ſkin and tongue dry and parched. Had this day Infus. Tamarind. cum Senna, which operated three times: Rice-water with tamarinds boiled in it for drink, and ſeveral glaſſes of Madeira wine.

On the fifth, looks more unpromiſing; pulſe quick, ſmall, and very frequent; ſkin dry and parched; conſtant jactation and uncovering his breaſt. At night, very indiſtinct; moans much in a wild and altered tone of voice; and refuſes his wine and drinks.—Applic. Emplaſt. Veſicator. inter ſcapulas, et habeat Hauſt. Anodyn. h. ſ.

The ſixth; had ſweated much laſt night, but without any relief. General appearance no better; ſtill refuſes his wine and drinks, but takes ſome at times when much preſſed. Is perfectly reſtleſs and delirious; attempting often to get out of his cot. Sleeps, but moans greatly; and when awake,

awake, feems much diftreffed. Pulfe very frequent, contracted, and irregular. At night cannot be got to fwallow any thing.—Applic. Cataplafmata cum Sinap. aliquantum pedibus.

On the feventh, pulfe feeble and irregular. Has had a ftool both yefterday and this morning. Extremities cold; cannot be got to fwallow any thing; refpiration quick and interrupted; cadaverous fmell; voids urine and fæces infenfibly: by all which a fpeedy diffolution was to be expected; and this accordingly took place about five o'clock P. M.

The fervant of the mefs, a ftout young lad, who had all along attended Lieutenant R., about eight days after his mafter's death was attacked with the fame difeafe. He had been obferved drooping for a day or two, before he made any complaint, but denied there was any thing the matter with him. When he was forced to make known his ailment, he complained only of pains in his limbs, want of appetite, and uneafinefs at the pit of his ftomach. He was vomited with tartar emetic folution * in the forenoon, and found himfelf better

* Solutio Tartritis Antimon.

ter towards night. Next day, he thought himſelf much eaſier, and continued to go about the decks, though his pulſe was ſomewhat quick and ſmall; but the fever returned again in the evening. A few ſmall doſes of antimonial ſolution had been given him through the day, and procured ſome ſtools.

On the morning of the third, pulſe ſtill ſmall and frequent; ſkin hot, and breathing quickened.—Capiat Pulv. Cort. Peruv. ʒſs. quatuor indies.

The fourth, complaints the ſame. No remiſſion yeſterday; tongue much furred; pulſe ſmall, and very frequent. Capiat ſtatim, Pulv. Sal. Nitri, gr. xv.; Tart. Antimon. gr. i., in Aq. fontan. ℥ij. After this, he vomited much green ſtuff, and had a remiſſion in the afternoon. Cont. Cortex Peruv. ad ʒi. quatuor indies.

The fifth, all his ſymptoms aggravated. A number of angry-looking puſtules this day broke out about his lips. Pulſe regular and free; ſays he throws up his drinks, which have been barley-water, or Infuſ. Althææ with tamarinds: This to be changed for weak tea. Has had a ſtool every day, and ſeveral after the laſt emetic. To take his bark in Julap. Salin.

The

The ſixth, general appearance the ſame as yeſterday. Tongue covered with a black dry cruſt; ſkin dry and parched. Cont. Cortex, and to have Madeira and water for drink *ad libitum.*

The ſeventh. This morning, ſymptoms ſtill more aggravated; only his pulſe is fuller: ſays he throws up the Madeira and water. To be changed again for the weak tea, cold; and to have a glaſs of claret, unmixed, five or ſix times a-day. Countenance retains a natural appearance, and the eruption about his mouth keeps out. Sleeps much; and when awoke, ſeems ſtartled, and requires ſome time to recollect himſelf, and give pertinent anſwers; but is otherwiſe free of delirium. Paſſes at times both urine and fæces inſenſibly. Cont. Cortex et Vin. rubr. At night, pulſe continues regular, but quick and feeble; is not ſenſible of his want of drink, but takes it when offered him; ſtill retains the bark on his ſtomach.—Capiat omni quartâ horâ ad ʒi. in Julap. Salin.

The eighth. This morning, looks worſe; is more inſenſible and oppreſſed; breathing very quick; ſtrong throbbing pulſation of the temporal arteries, and a few drops of blood have iſſued from his noſtril; ſtill he is ſenſible at times, and has regular

regular paſſage of his belly. Continues to take his wine and bark. Applic. Emplaſtra Veſicator. brachiis et cruribus. About eight at night, his pulſe became ſo low and feeble, as hardly to be felt at the wriſt; his hands and feet rather cold, with a cold ſweat over his breaſt. In this ſtate, he lay for a conſiderable time in a kind of ſtupor, without paying any attention to what was ſaid to him, and appeared ſo low as to render it doubtful whether he might ſurvive till morning. After ſome hours he began to recover a little; a degree of heat ſpread itſelf over his limbs, and he was able to ſwallow ſome warm wine. By next morning, a criſis was plainly diſtinguiſhable, by a fuller pulſe, and ſofter ſkin, with a redneſs and moiſture on the edges of his tongue. From this period the fever abated gradually, and he recovered ſtrength enough to walk the decks in leſs than a fortnight, with the aſſiſtance of bark and wine, and light diet.

Theſe two appear to have been fevers of the Bilious Remitting kind, pretty diſtinctly marked; and the event of the laſt caſe affords a preſumption,

tion, that in Lieutenant R's, where the early remiſſions were more perfect, bark might have had good effects. But as the fever ſpread no farther in the ſhip, we had no further means of putting it to proof. Had the diſeaſe once got among the troops under the deck, we had no reaſon to ſuppoſe it could have ſoon ſubſided, or that many would not have been cut off by it; but the ſeamens' ſick-birth being on the open deck, ſecured them from this danger. It continued to prevail in the tranſports with the 42d and 98th regiments for a conſiderable period; and a number both of officers and men, fell a ſacrifice to it; while it deſerves to be remarked, that all the troops and ſhips' companies who were encamped upon the beach, or on the dry and firm ſoil near it, have continued perfectly healthy.

After a tedious and painful paſſage of many weeks, ariſing from calms and exceſſive heats in recroſſing the Line, with ſhort allowance of both water and proviſions, and a conſtant current ſetting us to the weſtward, out of our courſe, the whole fleet came to anchor in the Bay of Moribat, on the coaſt of Arabia Felix, without the Straits of Babelmandel, in Lat. 17° 30′ North.

On this paſſage, the fleet in general ſuffered comparatively little from ſickneſs or diſeaſe, except thoſe ſhips which brought the fever from Johanna. After the two caſes of it in the Manilla, we had only a few ſlight and ſhort fevers among the ſoldiers, from expoſure to the exceſſive heats, attended with a redundancy of bile, diſtinguiſhed by a loaded yellow tongue, headach, oppreſſion and ſickneſs at ſtomach. A gentle vomit, followed by a purgative, if given early, was generally ſufficient for removing the ſymptoms, or a repetition of them, if neceſſary, was conſtantly ſucceſsful. It took on no regular type or duration, where there exiſted no infectious miaſmata to combine with it.

What contributed to the healthineſs of this part of the voyage, was the complete waſhing and cleaning of the ſhips and ſoldiers' births while they were emptied at Johanna; while the bedding, linen, and every part of the clothing, underwent the ſame proceſs on ſhore; ſo that not only did the people return to them in good health; but the ſhips themſelves, and every part of the clothing, were in much better condition than when we firſt embarked.

On

On this paſſage we loſt the ſhip's maſter, who was found one morning dead in his cabin, moſt probably from an over-doſe of brandy, as he had no known complaint.

The air at Moribat appears to be very pure and dry. The heat at this ſeaſon was great, both with ſea and land breeze. The ſoil is rocky and ſandy, without vegetation, or the leaſt veſtige of tree or ſhrub within view of the ſhore. About a mile back, the land riſes in a high precipitous craggy ridge, which faces the coaſt for a conſiderable length. Behind this, it is more elevated, and vegetation much greater. No water was found here, except a little, very brackiſh, near the ſhore. The inhabitants of a fiſhing village, from which the bay derives its name, bring all they uſe from wells ſeveral miles inland, on the backs of camels. Of courſe our ſupply here was very ſcanty; nor could we procure any article of freſh proviſions, except a few lean goats; nor any vegetable, but ſome preſerved dates. Fiſh, in great plenty and variety, were indeed procured in the Bay; in ſo much, that a ſingle draught of a ſhip's net, would ſometimes procure ſufficient to ſerve for a meal to the whole fleet.

Before we left this ftation, the fevers which had been brought from Johanna had entirely fubfided in all the fhips, and no new difeafes were caught by communication with this fhore. A number of our fhip's crew and foldiers, indeed, got bowel diforders, from eating too plentifully of the fifh, fometimes not in the foundeft ftate of prefervation. Similar diforders were imputed, by fome of the furgeons, to ufing the brackifh water; but it was clearly owing to the fifh diet.

The complaint was attended with griping, purging, and an inflated belly; very often with rufhes and efflorefcences on the fkin: and our people had more of it after going to fea than while at anchor, from attempting to cure and preferve the fifh, by rubbing them with wafhed falt from the pickle tubs, and drying them in the fun,—a procefs in which they were not very fuccefsful; but they ate them imperfectly cured, rather than the falt beef and pork, fo long as they lafted. A purge or two, with plentiful dilution, and abftaining from the fifh, was fufficient for removing all the diforder. The fleet were, in a manner, tide-bound in this bay for fome weeks, by the current fetting towards the Straits. As foon as it began fomewhat to abate,

abate, the Monmouth, Hero and Iſis attempted the paſſage to Bombay, working as much in-ſhore along the coaſt as they could, where the current was ſlacker. The only other ſhip that at this time attempted the paſſage, was the Manilla, and ſhe was enabled to keep up with the men of war, by the advantage ſhe had in her leſs draught of water, whereby ſhe could work her courſe much more in-ſhore. In leſs than three weeks we made the harbour of Bombay, and the other diviſion of the fleet, which had been left at Moribat, arrived in a ſhort time after. Among the troops ſcorbutic diatheſis had begun again to manifeſt itſelf, and ſome who had ſuffered much by fluxes formerly, were again attacked, but not in the dyſenteric form. Of ſuch caſes, two were loſt on this part of the paſſage.

At this time a ſoldier's wife, of a fair complexion, and delicate habit, was, without any known cauſe, attacked with inflammation in one of her eyes, attended with dimneſs of ſight, and pain over that ſide of the head. A thick ſpeck, of a dead white, ſoon appeared on the lower edge of the cornea, but, what was rather curious, was not fixed exactly to one place, but roſe higher or fell lower at different times of the day. In the forenoon, it was ſometimes ſo high as to obſtruct the paſſage of light through the pupil entirely: in the evening it was often lower than even the cornea lucida. At other times it was more fixed to a ſpot, but increaſed in ſize; was more painful in the forenoon, and became eaſier, and diminiſhed towards night. Doſes of cooling phyſic and saturnine lotions gave little or no relief. The means of topical bleeding were wanting, and her habit was too delicate to admit of any conſiderable evacuation of blood from the arm. A bliſter over the temple and forehead of the affected ſide ſoon relieved the pain, and diminiſhed the general inflammation; and the ſpeck gradually diſappeared, and left the eye perfectly ſound. As we advanced to the northward, the coaſt conſiſted of a dead flat, covered with a barren white ſand, as far inland as the eye could reach; and we were always within view of the ſhore, and generally very near it. Whether this caſe of ophthalmia might have been occaſioned by a fine drift ſand from the beach, or the uncommon glare of light reflected from it, I did not then conjecture; but from what I ſaw afterwards in India, I rather ſuſpect the latter

ter. These were cases of nyctolopia, or perfect vision only in the evening, and were most common in subjects who had been long in the country. The eye appeared sound, but they had commonly pain in the head, saw very imperfectly in the day-time, and the pupil appeared contracted to a perfect point; whereas, in the twilight, it was much more dilated, and vision was much better. After refreshing for about ten days at Bombay, the Manilla, with the men of war, and part of the India ships, sailed again for Madras, which we reached in five weeks, and landed all the troops and stores from the ships. Thus finishing, in exactly eleven months, a tedious and suffering passage from England. In the latter periods of this, I was not furnished with the number of deaths among the troops as they happened in the ship; but from the account of the hospital mates, and the officers returns, I learned, that out of the two companies embarked, with some occasional fillings up from the other ships as the numbers decreased, they had lost, upon the whole, 75 men. Forty from fevers; 18 from dysenteric flux; and the remainder, from scurvy and cachexy. Of the ship's company, we lost the lieutenant and one seaman from fever; one feaman from flux combined with fcurvy ; and the mafter, accidentally. From the beft accounts I could procure, the deaths in fome of the India fhips and tranfports had been in a fimilar proportion. In others of the larger tranfports, and in the men of war, the loffes were greatly inferior.

By ftating a comparifon between the mortality among the feamen and the troops in this fhip, nothing more is intended than to point out the good effect of the pure and free air, in which the former were kept above deck, both through the night and day, over that in which the latter were below the hatches, for preferving the health, and in refifting contagion and difeafe at fea.

On this fubject, the following obfervations may not be irrelevant.

Since the date of this expedition, many and great reforms have taken place in the modes of fea-victualling, and in the fupplies for the fick. Much more attention has been paid to cleanlinefs, and to the means for correcting foul air in fhips ; and for refifting contagion by fumigation, &c. How far thefe these meliorations have been extended to the transport service, I am ignorant. In the manner in which those employed on our expedition were fitted up, with standing platforms for the soldiers' beds, many of them were rendered impracticable. In the latter part of the voyage, we became so sensible of this in the Manilla, that these were all cleared away, and the soldiers supplied with hammocks. The ship was also much overcrowded for her size, whereby all these things are rendered tenfold more difficult than where there is more room. With regard to sea-scurvy, reports and accounts have been published, as if this had been cured at sea, by lime or citron juice, lemon rob, nitre dissolved in vinegar, nitric acid, &c. all which I would suspect to be rather something of the hyperbolical. But there is a plan for this purpose recommended by a Mr Young of the Navy, which, from its practicability, and perfect conformity to known and established principles, is highly deserving of attention, and of being recorded in such a publication as this. It proceeds upon the well known fact, that nothing more is necessary for the cure of this disease in any situation where there is a tolerably pure air, than,—not dead and dried,

dried, but fresh vegetable diet, greens or roots, in sufficient quantity. To be sure, we cannot have a kitchen-garden at sea, and a short and scanty crop of greens can only be raised on board a ship; but beans and pease, and barley, and other seeds, can be carried in any quantity; and as Mr Young has very justly stated any kind of esculent seeds brought under the malting or vegetating process, are converted into the state of a growing plant, with the vital principle in full activity throughout the germ and pulp: and if eaten in this state without any sort of preparation, except that of separating or rejecting the husks, cannot fail to supply precisely what is wanted for the cure of scurvy, viz. fresh vegetable chyle. For this purpose, besides the articles already mentioned, which may all be employed, he gives the preference to *gram*, an East India grain, chiefly used in the feeding of horses. The malting process is to be performed in shallow frames of wood, constructed so as to preserve the water for successive operations; and a little experience will readily lead to the proper degrees of heat and moisture for conducting it successfully.

We

We have only further to obſerve, that in all long voyages, it ought to be our object, not only to find out and employ the moſt effectual means to prevent or cure this diſeaſe, as one that proves fatal by itſelf, but alſo to guard as far as poſſible againſt the taint; as that which never fails to give a fatal or malignant tendency to other diſorders incident to this way of life; as ulcers, fevers, fluxes, &c.; and, in order to this, our preventive plan ought to commence from the firſt day on which the ſailing ſtock of freſh vegetables, and ſhip's beer, is expended: Since, from many examples it appears, that much greater ſucceſs is likely to attend our endeavours in this way, than by reſerving them for the period in which the marks of ſcorbutic diatheſis begin to manifeſt themſelves. In other words, every healthy ſeaman carries with him to ſea a certain quantity or proportion of antiſcorbutic humours. The ſtock may be preſerved, if huſbanded with care; but cannot, in that ſituation be eaſily recovered, if once it is ſuffered to run down.

INDIA DISEASES.

SPASMODIC CHOLERA,—THE CRAMP,—OR, MORI DE CHIEN.

IN the beginning of the year 1782, the Hero, Monmouth, Iſis, and ſeveral of the King's tranſport ſhips, joined the fleet under Sir Edward Hughes at Madras. He had juſt returned from the capture of ſeveral Dutch ſettlements on the coaſt. The acceſſion of three ſhips of the line, gave activity to his preparations for further and more important conqueſts, when the arrival of *our* old acquaintance, the French Admiral Souffrain, with twelve ſail of line of battle ſhips, cut out for us other employment, and put an end to our dreams of bloodleſs victories and further acquiſitions.

The firſt meeting between the fleets took place to the ſouthward of Madras, and ended in a drawn battle. On this occaſion, I was on board the Iſis, whoſe whofe furgeon was unable to act at the time; and on the return of the fleet, was appointed to do duty on board the Seahorfe 20 gun fhip.

In this ftation, I had the firft opportunity of becoming acquainted with this fatal and untractable India difeafe. Of the names here given to it, the two laft only were employed in the country. How far the firft may be ftrictly appropriate or fcientific, is fubmitted to the judgment and opinion of others.

On the 12th of April 1782, the day of Rodney's fplendid victory in the weft, a fecond meeting, and a battle of five hours continuance, took place between the fleets. But *fo* it did not end with us, but in hard blows and bruifes only. This happened fome way to the fouthward of Trincomalé; and was fought fo near the fhore, that both fleets came to anchor in the evening in the fame place where it had been contefted, fcarcely out of reach of gun-fhot from each other.

Here they both remained for more than a week, repairing damages, and looking at each other. The French fhips had fuffered leaft in action; they were the firft to put to fea; and offered us battle for a whole day in vain,—not from any

want

want of courage, either of the Admiral, or of the fleet, but blundering and mismanagement had tied up our hands. The strength of the two fleets had been nearly equal; and whatever might be reported in gazettes at home, *we* certainly claimed no victory. When the French had left the coast clear, the British fleet made sail for Trincomalé, and anchored in Back Bay. An hospital was established on shore for the sick and wounded; but the Seahorse being for some time detached on service within the Great Bay, I had but few opportunities of seeing what was going on in it. Wounds, ulcers, and burns from the explosion of gunpowder, made up the bulk of surgical cases: Fluxes and fever diseases, the chief part of the remainder. The mort de chien, or cramp, I was also informed by the attending surgeons, had been very frequent and fatal among the seamen, both at the hospital and in some of the ships, particularly in the Hero and Superb.

The Seahorse did not join the fleet in Back Bay till the 14th of May, when the disease had become much less frequent, nor had we any men attacked with it till the 21st of June.

Previous

Previous to this, our ſhip's company had been very healthy, though they had been a good deal expoſed and employed in ſevere duty within the great harbour; only a few ſlight fluxes had appeared, and which we imputed to the water at Fort Oſnaburg, which is ſomewhat brackiſh, and apt to occaſion bowel diſorders. One, however, turned out differently, and ended in a way which gave me much uneaſineſs. This caſe is added after the liver-diſeaſes, with a view to ſhew the neceſſity of making ourſelves well acquainted with the peculiarities and ſymptoms of diſeaſes that are varied by the influence of climate, in order to practiſe with ſafety or ſucceſs in a foreign country.

The weather was at this period rough and bluſtering. A conſtant land-wind, blowing ſometimes in guſts and ſqualls, and without any ſea-breeze, had already ſet in. A ſtrong and conſtant land-wind prevails during the months of July and Auguſt, along the whole eaſtern ſide of the coaſt; but here it ſets in much earlier; and by coming over a country thickly covered with buſhes, trees and underwood, feels much colder. This is never heated by the ſun ſo much as a bare and ſandy

ſoil;

ſoil; but when rain or dews fall, a copious and quick evaporation takes place, whereby the air becomes loaded with moiſture, cooled down to a conſiderable degree.

Early in the morning of the 21ſt of June, we had two men ſiezed with the mort de chien, both of whom we loſt in a few hours; and in the courſe of the two following days, three more in the ſame complaint, without meeting with one fortunate caſe. To the 25th, when we ſailed for Negapatam, we had three new caſes of the ſame kind; all of whom were ſaved, but two of them with great difficulty. Beſides theſe, we had ſeveral others which were of a nature conſiderably different, being evidently combined with bilious colluvies in the firſt paſſages; a circumſtance not at all diſcoverable, either in the firſt five caſes that ended fatally, nor in two of the others that ſucceeded. All theſe were found to be much more tractable, eaſily removed, and attended with but little danger.

In every one of the eight caſes, the ſymptoms were ſo much alike, both in order and degree, that a deſcription of any one would anſwer almoſt equally well for every other. Any difference that took

took place was in the ſuddenneſs of the attack, or the rapidity with which the ſymptoms ſucceeded each other. In all of them the diſeaſe began with a watery purging, attended with ſome teneſmus, but with little or no griping. This always came on ſome time in the night, or early towards morning, and continued ſome hours before any ſpaſms were felt; or theſe were confined to the toes and feet; and ſlight affections of this kind being very common in the country, the patients ſeldom mentioned them till they began to be more ſevere, and extended to the legs or thighs. This purging ſoon brought on great weakneſs, coldneſs of the extremities, and a remarkable paleneſs, ſinking and lividity of the whole countenance. Some at this period had ſome nauſea and retching to vomit, but brought up nothing bilious. In a ſhort time the ſpaſms began to affect the muſcles of the thighs, abdomen and thorax, and laſtly they paſſed to thoſe of the arms, hands and fingers; but I never ſaw, then or afterwards, thoſe of the neck, face or back at all affected. The rapidity with which theſe ſpaſms ſucceeded the firſt attack, and their ſeverity, eſpecially as affecting the muſcles of the thorax and abdomen, denoted in general the degree of danger in the cafe. The affection is not as in tetanus confined to a fingle mufcle, or to a certain clafs of mufcles only. Neither does it, as in the fpafmus clonicus, move and agitate the members. It is a fixed cramp in the belly of the mufcle, which is gathered up into a hard knot, with excruciating pain. In a minute or two this relaxes, is again renewed, or the affection paffes to others, leaving the miferable fufferer hardly an interval of eafe; and, laftly, it paffes from one fet to another; from thofe of the inferior extremity to thofe on the upper parts, leaving the former free. The patients complain much of the pain of thefe cramps; think they obtain fome relief from friction of the parts, and cry to their companions to rub them hard. As the difeafe proceeded, the countenance became more and more pale, wan and dejected; the eyes became funk, hollow, and furrounded with a livid circle. The pulfe became more feeble, and fometimes fank fo much, as not to be felt at the wrift, in two or three hours after the fpafms came on. But fo long as it could be felt, it was but little altered in frequency. If the fpafms happened to intermit, it would fometimes rife a little, and the countenance

affume

aſſume a better look. The tongue was generally white, and more or leſs furred towards the root; and the patients had all great thirſt, or rather a ſtrong deſire for cold drinks; but there was no headach or affection of the ſenſorium commune throughout.

The coldneſs of the extremities, which was perceptible from the very firſt, continued to increaſe, and ſpread over the whole body, but with no moiſture on the ſkin, till the ſeverity of the pain and ſpaſms forced out a clammy ſweat, which ſoon became profuſe. The hands now began to put on a ſtriking and peculiar appearance. The nails of the fingers became livid, and bent inwards; the ſkin of the palms became white, bleached, and wrinkled up into folds, as if long ſoaked in cold water; the effect, no doubt, of the profuſe cold ſweat, which is one of the moſt pernicious and fatal ſymptoms of the diſeaſe; both from the effect it has in ſuch a climate, of exhauſting the ſtrength, and in abſtracting heat from the ſyſtem. In ſome of the preſent caſes, and in many others after this, we had recoveries from the ſevereſt degrees of ſpaſmodic affection; even where the pulſe had been for hours completely loſt at the wriſt, and the body perfectly cold; but never of any who had these profuse cold clammy sweats, and where the hands had put on this appearance.

All this while the purging continued frequent, and exhibited nothing but a thin watery matter or mucus. In many, the stomach became at last so irritable, that nothing could be got to rest upon it; but every thing that was drunk, was spouted up immediately, without straining or retching. The countenance and extremities became livid; the pulsations of the heart more quick, frequent and feeble; the breathing began to become laborious and panting; and, in fine, the whole powers of life fell under such a great and speedy collapse, as to be soon beyond the power of recovery. In this progression, the patient remained from three to five or six hours from the accession of the spasms; seldom longer. These began at last to abate, but with more internal oppression, great jactation, panting and gasping for breath; from the diminished action of the respiratory organs: for there were no marks of oppression or effusion on the lungs; and the motion of the heart, so long as it could be felt, became more and more quick and irregular, till

till death came at laſt to the relief of the miſerable ſufferer.

Some time before that event took place, the ſpaſms, gradually abating, left the ſufferers entirely; and ſo much poſſeſſion of their faculties did they retain, that they would continue to talk ſenſibly to their meſſmates, to the laſt moment of their life, even when the whole body had become perfectly cold, and all pulſation at the heart had ceaſed for a long time to be diſtinguiſhable.

A variety of opinions were entertained about the proximate and exciting cauſes of this diſeaſe; ſome imputing it to the influence of cold and damp winds, eſpecially the land-winds of the night *,

* The prevailing winds along the coaſt of Coromandel, from the middle of July to the end of Auguſt, are from the land; and they blow often ſtrong; feel hot, ſultry and parching; have much effect in checking perſpiration, during even the great heat of the day; render the ſkin hot and dry, with an uneaſy ſenſation in the noſtrils, lips and eyes; render the reſpiration unpleaſant, and ſometimes occaſion nauſea and ſickneſs at ſtomach. At Trincomalé, the land-wind ſets in earlier in the ſeaſon; and owing to the circumſtances formerly noticed, gives rather an uneaſy ſenſation of coldneſs. On the coaſt, the ſoil is generally bare, dry and ſandy, which affects the winds blowing over it very differently.

in giving a ſudden check to perſpiration; whereby ſomething deleterious, that ought to have been thrown off by the ſkin, was retained in the ſyſtem; and without doubt the ſtate of the weather, while the fleet were at Trincomalé, and the circumſtance of almoſt all the attacks being in the night-time, gave ſome countenance to this opinion. That which prevailed among the older ſurgeons on the ſtation, led, as I know it was, by a deſervedly great and high authority at Madras, but taken from a haſty and imperfect letter on the ſubject, ſtill more looſely and imperfectly taken up and underſtood;—aſcribed the proximate cauſe to the action of diſeaſed bile in the firſt paſſages: conſidering it in the ſame light as the true Cholera Morbus of the ſyſtematic writers.

Others, again, by obſerving it to prevail more in certain ſeaſons than in others, or in certain tracks and ſpots, or in ſhips anchored in the ſame line of direction, while others, placed at no great diſtance, kept entirely free from it, imputed the complaint to ſome delcterious exhalations paſſing through the atmoſphere, in certain tracks and lines of direction, in the manner of the *ſimmoon* or *ſamiel* blaſts of the Deſart.

It

It was a common opinion among the ſurgeons, that it attacked moſt readily the moſt irregular and worſt clothed men; but in the Seahorſe, ſome of the beſt clothed and orderly men in the ſhip were affected with it.

In whatever the proximate cauſe might conſiſt, two diſtinct and ſeemingly oppoſite affections were obſervable at the ſame time. Great debility and irritability of the whole alimentary canal, with impaired action of the heart and arteries, along with a violent increaſed action of the voluntary muſcles; but how connected as cauſe and effect, or depending both of them on ſome particular affection of the nervous ſyſtem, may be difficult to explain. The moſt ſtriking and alarming ſymptom is, the great and ſudden proſtration of ſtrength, and depreſſion of the powers concerned in carrying on the circulation and in maintaining the vital functions, without being the effect of great depletion, or of *exhauſted excitement*, as the Brunonians ſpeak; for the evacuations are, from the firſt, a thin watery mucus in trifling quantity. Little or nothing is ejected by any retchings that happen; and it is obſervable from the very firſt, before the ſyſtem has ſuffered much from the ſtimulus of pain, or the ſeverity of the ſpaſms. In the Seahorſe, it attacked ſome remarkably robuſt, powerful and muſcular men, who had been in perfect health immediately before. Neither in all our claſs of bad and fatal caſes, did there appear any marks of bilious colluvies, either in the colour of the ejected matters, the ſtate of the abdomen, or in the appearance of the tongue, eyes and urine. There was neither pain nor griping, nor ſoreneſs or tenderneſs on preſſing the belly. We had indeed another ſet of caſes, where the preſence of this was diſtinguiſhable by all theſe characters; but theſe were of a far ſlighter nature, and none of them turned out any way untractable or fatal.

By this time I had both learned the general opinion about the diſeaſe, and ſeen the ſource of it in the letter mentioned; imputing the proximate cauſe in a general way to the action of putrid and diſeaſed bile in the firſt paſſages; and the influence of certain occaſional or exciting cauſes, putting it into motion and activity. But I had met with a caſe on our paſſage from Madras, which, in perfect ignorance of all theſe theories, and even of the name of ſuch a diſorder, I had cured by opium alone, and I determined to follow what I thought

thought the guide of experience. A ſtout healthy man was ſuddenly ſeized with the ſymptoms of this diſeaſe, which ſoon became ſevere. The ſpaſms appearing the moſt alarming and urgent part of the complaint, and the patient being in the vigour of life, and of uncommon muſcular ſtrength, four grains of ſolid opium in two pills, were given him on his firſt complaint, and two or three tea ſpoonfuls of a mixture of equal parts of laudanum and ether were rubbed into the pit of his ſtomach. In half an hour the ſpaſms not abating, his pulſe becoming weak, his heat diminiſhing, and his countenance pale and ſunk, after fomenting his legs with cloths rung out of warm ſea-water, and rubbing them well afterwards with dry flannel, four grains more of opium were given him in a ſmall glyſter. In about two hours after this, the ſpaſms began to abate; he recovered more heat, and looked better. An ounce and a half of Glauber's ſalt was given him, to counteract the aſtringent effects of ſo much opium; after which he vomited a little, was well covered up in his hammock; ſoon grew hot, and ſweated ſome. The cramps left him, and he recovered the natural firmneſs of his pulſe, and a natural look; ſlept well through the night, and

was

was perfectly well the next day, exeept a watery loofenefs, which continued for a few days after.

Recollecting the fuccefs of this cafe, our firft patient at Trincomalé, had, on his firft complaint, four grains of opium in two pills, and his ftomach was well rubbed with laudanum and ether. Sometime after this, a laxative glyfter was adminiftered; and he was put into a warm bath of fea-water, where he continued about fifteen minutes. On coming out of this, he was well rubbed and covered up in bed, and had for drink warm wine, well mulled with fpices. The fpafms did not abate, and his ftools continued thin, watery and frequent. The laxative glyfter, and warm bathing were both repeated without any good effect. A cold clammy fweat came out, and he died in about four hours after the cramps came on.

The event of this cafe unfettled my opinion as to the efficacy of opium, and threw me back to the authority already mentioned. I had heard much of latent and lurking bile, as the general fource of India difeafe, and refolved to feek for, and hunt it out by the means employed by others, viz. repeated fmall dofes of Sal. Glauber in Aq. Menth. Pip. and fharpened with a very fmall proportion of

Emetic

Emetic Tartar, ſuch as an eight part of a grain to each doſe, with a view to quicken the operation of the ſalts downwards *. This plan was accordingly tried with our next patient. He threw up a very ſmall quantity of greeniſh-coloured bile, and the ſolution operated much downwards : but without any relief or diſcharge of bilious matter. I next gave him three grains of opium diſſolved in a ſmall mucilaginous glyſter, and as ſoon as it ſettled in his bowels, he was put into the warm bath ; after which he was well covered up in bed, with warmed cloths conſtantly applied to his ſtomach and limbs ; and he drank hot wine, mulled with ſpices. No relief appearing to follow theſe meaſures, a warm purgative glyſter was given him, but was followed by no bilious diſcharge. No vomiting continued after the firſt exhibition of the purgative ; but a repetition of it, to ſee if any bile lurked ſtill in the ſtomach, and could be ſolicited downwards,

* How ſuch a laxative had ever come into uſe, I do not now conceive. None could have been leſs ſuited to the ſtate of the diſeaſe, in any form in which it occurred. Both of the articles are by far too irritating, and debilitating in their operation, to be adapted to any of the bowel diſorders of India, and they were accordingly ſoon entirely diſcarded from uſe.

downwards, brought on continued retching, and he threw up after this every thing he drank, till his death, which happened in five hours after his firſt complaint. In neither of theſe two patients, had the opiate the ſmalleſt effect, either in reſtraining the purging, or in abating the ſpaſmodic affection. At this time, by deſire of the captain, we were viſited by the admiral's ſurgeon. The flag-ſhip had been the ſevereſt ſufferer by the diſeaſe; and this gentleman diſapproved entirely of the uſe of opiates, and recommended the employment of purgatives;—the purgative antimonial ſolution, caſtor oil, rhubarb and calomel, with purgative glyſters; and what was of really more worth than all of them, warm ſtimulating cordials, and the application of heat in every poſſible way.

This plan was accordingly followed in the two ſucceeding caſes, one of them ill at the time; all with the ſame ill ſucceſs. One of them died in ſeven, and the other in eight hours illneſs.

In the caſe of our fifth patient, after giving the ſolution, till it operated both ways a little, and he had been in the warm bath, I had recourſe again to opium. Two grains were firſt given him, and repeated in an hour, with the addition to each of

ſix

ſix grains of camphor, and as much aromatic powder *, made up into a bolus. He was covered up in bed, and had warm tea, made ſtrong with arrack, for drink. After this, he ſweated ſome; his heat and pulſe were reſtored in ſome degree; his countenance aſſumed a better look, and the ſpaſms had nearly left him. But his breathing became catching and laborious; and he had a ſtrong craving for cold drink, which, however, was withheld from him, and he was half-forced to drink warm wine, mulled with ſpiceries. Heat was applied to his body in every poſſible way; but nothing had any further effect in recovering this, or in raiſing his pulſe; and he died in five hours after the ſpaſms had reached the abdomen. This patient was evidently dozed with the opium, and afforded the only inſtance where this effect was perceptible from it.

The ſymptoms in the caſe of our ſixth patient differed in no reſpect from any of the foregoing, except that the ſpaſms were never ſo general or ſevere. His pulſe was at one time ſo weak, as not to

* Pulv. Aromat. *Ph. Lond.*

to be felt at the wrift ; but after being in the bath for twenty minutes, it could be again diftinguifhed, and never became fo quick as in the advanced ftage in the other patients. A part of the notes relating to his cafe having been loft, I cannot fay what was done for him in the firft inftance ; but the fequel begins with obferving, That he had all along complained of fome pain and confufion in his head ;—that the pupils of his eyes were dilated. Some hours after being in the bath, his heat and pulfe returned in a tolerable degree, and the fpafms left him. A glyfter, with fome Ol. Ricin. was given him, and repeated again in the evening, without producing much difcharge. Next day, he ftill complained of weaknefs, confufion in his head, and the pupils ftill kept dilated. His pulfe was rather frequent, and his appetite was bad ; but he mentioned no other complaint. Wine and nourifhing diet was prefcribed for him, and he had fome dofes of calomel and James's powder at night. In this way, he lingered on to the tenth day from the firft attack, when he died in a low dozing ftupid ftate *.

Along

* See a fimilar inftance in the letter fubjoined. This was the only cafe I knew of, where the patient furvived the firft attack,

Along with the laſt caſe, we had two ſtrong and healthy ſeamen attacked in the night, in the uſual manner.

I had by this time begun to conclude, that the proximate cauſe of the diſeaſe was not to be ſought for in the ſtate of the bile, nor of any of the alvine ſecretions, and that without any reaſoning concerning this, our remedies ought to be directed more to obviate or remove the moſt urgent and dangerous ſymptoms,—to ſupport the *vires naturæ*; the circulation and heat in the external parts, and that evacuations were not to be urged any further than merely to clear the ſtomach and bowels once. Accordingly, our two patients had each, as ſoon as I was called in the morning, a ſingle doſe of the purgative ſolution. It only produced in one ſome retching, and brought away ſome phlegm. Both were put immediately into the bathing tubs, which were now kept ready for uſe. After remaining there for a quarter of an hour, they were well dried, and rubbed all over with

attack, and did not fully recover from the effects of the diſeaſe. This caſe appearing, by its termination, ſomewhat different from all the reſt, ſtood ſingle in the notes, and has been accordingly left out in the general enumeration.

with warm arrack, and well covered up in bed with warm blankets rolled up and laid along their fides and between their legs, with plenty of warm tea and arrack for drink. In an hour, the fpafms not abating, the coldnefs of the extremities, finking of the pulfe, and the finking and lividity of the countenance rather increafing; they were again put into the bath, and the fame courfe of frictions and covering up in bed repeated. One recovered his heat a little while in the bath, when he ate fome food, and his pulfe, which was fcarcely diftinguifhable before, could again be diftinctly felt at the wrift. He took, in two portions, after being covered up in bed, Sp. Minder. ℥i. *, Sp. Lavend. comp. ʒij., Aq. Fontan. et Arrack a ℥ij.. Fell foon into a warm foft fweat; recovered his ufual heat and firmnefs of pulfe, and was well next morning, except that he had a watery purging, which continued fome days, but went off under the ufe of mulled claret, and a dofe of caftor-oil. The other took, after coming out of the bath the fecond time, Ol. Menth. Pip. gtt. iij., Spt. Corn. Cervi

* Aq. Acetitis Ammoniæ, *Ph. Ed.*

Cervi gtt. lx. * in divided portions of rice-water, and afterwards warm tea and arrack for common drink. His pulfe, which had been completely gone at the wrift, did not return, but the fpafms had abated while in the bath. A cold fweat came out on his extremities, and every part of the body became perfectly cold; nor could the pulfe be diftinguifhed for two hours after this. His countenance became exceedingly wan, funk and livid. with general oppreffion, anxiety and jactation. He drank much of the warm tea with arrack; his pulfe began at laft to be felt, trembling at the wrift, and the fpafms gradually went off. He fell into a found fleep, and was next morning free from all complaint, except languor and weaknefs, fome pain of his head, and a watery loofenefs, which remained fome days; and for which only a dofe of rhubarb and calomel was prefcribed for him. Both thefe patients had, during the complaint, glyfters of plain rice-water warmed, two or three times thrown up, merely to fupply heat internally.

A feaman, who had been for fome days affected with a fevere flux, attended with griping, ftrain-

 ing,

* Aq. Carbon. Ammoniæ, *Ph. Ed.*

ing, mucous and bilious coloured ftools, and for which he had taken feveral evacuant medicines, was at this time attacked with the ufual fymptoms of the mort de chien. Two grains of opium were given him on its firft invafion. This in a fhort time carried off the fpafms, and his pulfe, which had began to fink, was reftored to the natural ftate. He fweated fome, flept well through the night, and was well next day, but low and weak, and his flux ftill remained unabated and of the fame appearance, but was removed for the time by the ordinary medicines; at leaft he had made no further complaint, or I had neglected to take any further account of him. But it foon after appeared it had not been cured; that the fource of it had been deeper in the fyftem, and that, from the beginning, it had been the liver-flux, though he had not at this time any pain in the fide. Symptoms of inflamed liver, however, foon took place, of which he was effectually cured under my care in Madras hofpital, by a mercurial courfe.

The cafes that appeared after this, were all of a different nature, much lefs fevere, and none turned out fatal. They were all of them combined with bilious accumulations, and in patients where this diathefis

diathefis was vifibly prefent at the time. There was a load and oppreffion about the ftomach ; the evacuations, both by ftool and vomiting, were bilious, and the purging was attended with griping rather than tenefmus. The countenance, in place of becoming pale and livid, was fallow, and the tongue and eyes tinged with a yellow colour ; the feet and legs were very apt to become cold, but the fpafms were never fevere, and did not advance beyond the legs and thighs. The difeafe was eafily and fafely cured in all thefe, by gentle laxatives, joined with aromatics, warm glyfters, warm wine, and cordial diet and drinks.

Upon the whole, the difeafe prefented itfelf under two diftinct and different forms, and required a treatment that behoved to embrace a confiderable variety.

In what might be taken as fimple and uncombined cafes, where no fymptoms of bilious colluvies were diftinguifhable, from the appearance of the ejected matters, or from the ftate of the abdomen, or the colour of the tongue, eyes and urine I came at laft to conclude, that all kinds of evacuants were not only ufelefs but hurtful ; and that they only tended to increafe the proftration of ſtrength, the ſinking of the pulſe, and ſeverity of the ſpaſms; which, in all ſuch caſes, formed the moſt dangerous and alarming part of the complaint; and although, in ſuch circumſtances, there was no contra-indication to the uſe of opiates; yet, unleſs they were given early, before much ſinking of the pulſe, and failure of the *vires naturæ* had come on, their effect was but tranſient or uncertain, or only trifling and temporary; ſo that no benefit was likely to be derived from them, unleſs when given on the firſt acceſſion, in full doſe, and joined with ſome ſtimulus that acts ſpeedily and powerfully; ſuch as hot and cordial ſpiritous tinctures, the aromatic oils, or the volatile alkali. That in all ſuch caſes, the ſpaſmodic affection was only to be conſidered as ſymptomatic, depending perhaps on ſome of theſe latent and inexplicable operations and ſympathies of the nervous ſyſtem, about which it is of little uſe to puzzle ourſelves in practice; and that we had little to do with the diſcuſſion of proximate or other cauſes, any further than to obviate or remove, by change of place or otherwiſe, ſuch as might be unfavourable to the main object, viz. that of ſupporting the ſtrength, reſtoring the activity of the moving powers, and the healthy action of the ſtomach and inteſtines, by ſuch means as experience teaches us, are beſt adapted to excite the vitality and action of theſe organs.

In caſes where the exiſtence of bilious colluvies and diſeaſed ſecretions was to be diſtinguiſhed, a good deal of purging was always neceſſary, with cordial diet and drinks, but opiates never.

About the middle of July 1782, I entered on duty at Madras hoſpital. Here, again, I had occaſion to ſee many more caſes of the mort de chien. It was frequent in the fleet in the month of Auguſt, and beginning of September, the ſeaſon at which the land-wind prevails on this part of the coaſt. We had ſome caſes in the hoſpital in the end of October, and in November, after the monſoon, but few in compariſon. Here the deaths were much fewer than on board the ſhips. Out of about twenty under my care, only three were loſt. In general, the caſes were milder than at Trincomalé. About a third were evidently connected with bilious colluvies; and in theſe, there was no great ſinking of the pulſe, or diminution of heat; and the ſpaſms were confined to the legs and feet: there was ſome fever, and the

 pulſe

pulſe was frequent as well as feeble. The tongue was commonly foul, and the countenance ſallow. The abdomen tumid, or tender to the touch, with more or leſs griping, and bilious diſcharges by ſtool.

Theſe all did well under the uſe of gentle purgatives and glyſters frequently repeated, ſuch as decoction of Manna, with Cream of Tartar *, Decoct. Tamarind. cum Senn. and plentiful dilution with rice-water, with Caſſia boiled in it. When part of the bile was thus carried off, we ſometimes employed thoſe that were more active, as Ol. Ricin: and when the ſtomach was very irritable, Rhub. and Calomel †, made into ſmall pills, ſtaid better on it than any thing we tried, procuring free ſtools with as little griping as any. The ſaline or more active purges we entirely laid aſide. When the patient appeared to be too much weakened by the uſe of laxatives, we intermitted them, and gave warm wine with ſpices; often punch or toddy, till the ſtrength was recruited; but we never employed opiates, or aſtringents. In this way, the bile was by degrees ſafely abſtracted. The feveriſhneſs

---

* Supertartris Potaſſæ. † Submurias Hydrargyri.

feveriſhneſs abated, the patient ſoon recovered ſtrength, and the natural tone of the ſtomach and inteſtines; but the ſtate of theſe behoved, for ſome time, to be well looked after. The caſes that terminated fatally were all exactly of the ſame kind as thoſe we had at Trincomalé. A watery purging, but without any appearance of bile in the diſcharges, always preceded the cramps. This was ſoon followed by a great ſinking of pulſe, pale and livid countenance, and coldneſs of the extremities. This appearance of countenance was ſometimes ſo remarkable, even before any cramps had come on, that in going round the hoſpital, I ſometimes obſerved it, and foretold the acceſſion of ſpaſms an hour or two before any were felt; and in one or two inſtances, the diſeaſe was prevented from getting its full length, and the ſymptoms eaſily removed by applications made at this early period. In ſuch caſes, our treatment was ſomewhat different from that practiſed on board the ſhips. Rubbing the ſtomach, legs and feet with flannel ſprinkled with warm arrack, fomentations with large pieces of blanket applied as extenſively as poſſible, without expoſing the body to the external air, were preferred to the warm-bath, and warm wine was given, made hot with *chillies*. Draughts, with Sp. Corn. Cerv., Lavender and Ol. Menth. Pip., made as ſtrong as the patient could poſſibly ſwallow them, were given frequently, and glyſters of plain warm water frequently thrown up. No evacuants of any kind, or opiates, were made uſe of. In this way, almoſt all of them were recovered, even in caſes where the ſymptoms were exceedingly ſevere and unpromiſing. The patients who died were ſoon after opened: In two, there was nothing uncommon with regard to ſymptoms; nor were any morbid appearances found on diſſection. There was no bilious accumulations found any where, and the internal organs were all in a ſound ſtate; only there was more water than natural in the pericardium, and the veſſels of the lungs, liver and meſentery, appeared to be very turgid and full of blood. In the following caſes, the circumſtances of diſeaſe, and appearances on diſſection were particular.

CASE.

John Holland, ſoldier in the 98th regiment, doing duty as marine, æt. 30., was received into the hoſpital about the latter end of July, with ſymptoms

ſymptoms of inflamed liver, attended, as uſual, with a flux, and ſhort dry cough. Towards the end, the flux had been accompanied with ſevere ſtraining and gripes felt in the lower part of his belly, which was ſore and tender to the touch; and blood commonly followed his ſtools.

His ſide was early bliſtered, and cooling laxatives were given him; after which he went through a courſe of mercury, which removed all his complaints, except the griping pains felt in the lower part of the belly. But theſe were effectually relieved by the application of a bliſter over the part, and he never paſſed blood with his ſtools after this. He was conſidered as convaleſcent from hepatitis, and was put upon ſoap and ſquill pills, with doſes of caſtor oil occaſionally, to relieve coſtiveneſs, (a common conſequent upon liver obſtruction, or inflammation imperfectly removed;) but in other reſpects he had no complaint, and he had nearly recovered his former appetite, ſtrength and fleſh. On the 30th of Auguſt, he had liberty to walk out of the hoſpital; ate a hearty dinner in the Black Town, and drank a good deal of ſpirits. He was ſeized in the evening with looſeneſs and gripes; and, by midnight, ſevere cramps

in

in his legs and feet began to come on, and his countenance was pale and livid. Such was the account brought by the attendant of the ward, who received directions to administer some glysters, and a gentle laxative infusion of senna and tamarinds. On visiting him a few hours afterwards, I found his pulse scarcely to be felt at the wrist; his eyes sunk and hollow; his whole countenance livid; his hands and fingers contracted by the spasms, with the nails livid and bent inwards; the whole body perfectly cold, with great jactation, panting and gasping for breath. From his messmates I learned he had drank several times of cold water through the night; a fatal piece of imprudence in such complaints. All the ordinary remedies were employed for his recovery, but without effect, and he died early in the forenoon.

On opening his body in the evening, we found marks of inflammation, and even that some degree of suppuration had taken place in two or three places on the surface of the liver, though all had been healed up. Large cells, of a white colour, but containing no matter or fluid, penetrated to the depth of a quarter of an inch, in certain spots or patches of some extent; and over these

theſe places the covering membrane was thickened, puffy and white. In many places it adhered to the diaphragm and ſide; but its ſubſtance, when cut into, preſented every where a natural appearance; nor was it in any part, or the gall-bladder preternaturally large. The meſenteric veſſels were turgid, eſpecially towards the lower part of the ilium, and the glands enlarged. This enlargement of the glands was more remarkable upon the rectum. The coats of this gut were much inflamed and thickened. The diameter of the canal was in ſome places much contracted; the internal coat ſpongy and ulcerous in many portions, and, in ſome ſpots, had even a gangrenous look. Where the ilium enters the colon, there were ſimilar affections, but in a much inferior degree. The colon appeared to be pretty ſound, except that the glands of the meſocolon were enlarged and hard.

About four ounces of water were contained in the pericardium; and two ſoft polypous concretions adhered to the left ventricle of the heart.

The right lobe of the lungs adhered almoſt every where to the diaphragm and ſide; but there

was

was neither inflammation nor ulceration in any part of its fubftance.

This cafe of mort de chien feems to have been excited by topical irritation; and there were no marks of bilious colluvies, or that bile had been any way concerned. But it furnifhes a ferious caution againft irregularity and intemperance in fuch a country as India; it marks the ftrong difpofition to inflammatory difeafe of the abdominal vifcera, and the rapidity with which it proceeds to a gangrenous termination there.

CASE.

John Giggs, feaman, a young man belonging to the Magnanime, was in the other divifion of the hofpital for an ulcer on his leg, and was of a weak and reduced habit. On the 21ft of November, he firft complained of a purging, with fome gripes and ftraining, which, he faid, had affected him only for two days. Pulfe fomewhat quick. Tongue foul. The gentleman who prefcribed for him, ordered him a gentle vomit in the evening, and through the night and next day fmall dofes of Glauber falts, in divided portions, diffol-

ved

ved in rice-water, made hot with Spir. Menth. Pip.

On the 22d, he was attacked with ſpaſms in his limbs, though not at all ſevere. Pulſe ſmall and quick; countenance pale and ſunk; general pain and ſome ſpaſms in the abdominal muſcles. Belly rather tenſe and retracted, than tumid or full. He was ſuppoſed now to have that terrible diſeaſe the mort de chien, and latent and lurking bile at the bottom of it; and ſo a repetition of the Glauber ſalts, with a grain of emetic tartar in the whole ſolution, was preſcribed for him in divided doſes. This produced many motions downwards, but brought away little, except diſcoloured watery ſtuff. Glyſters of plain rice-water were thrown up the rectum two or three times through the night, and he drank plentifully of warm rice-water with ſome nitre diſſolved in it.

On the morning of the 23d all his ſpaſms had left him; he had but little pain in the abdomen, and looked better. But he became much worſe in the afternoon; for, though he continued free from cramps, his pulſe was very weak and quick; his countenance pale, ſunk and dejected; and the heat,

heat, tenſion and retraction of the abdomen, were greater than ever, with much pain on preſſing the umbilical region. His extremities became cold; and he was ſomewhat delirious, with conſtant jactation and reſtleſſneſs; but had no vomiting or retching. On repeating the purging mixture, however, it was thrown up; but glyſters and fomenting the abdomen were ſubſtituted in place of it. Warm wine with ſpices were frequently given him; and a large bliſter was applied in the evening over the middle of the abdomen.

On the morning of the 24th, he was not relieved, he complained much of his belly and right ſide; and the proſtration of ſtrength was greater. Bliſter had riſen well: an opiate and ſome mulled wine were given him without any relief, and he died early in the forenoon.

On opening the body the following morning, the caput cœcum coli and about three inches of the colon were found in a completely mortified ſtate. On cutting into it, a putrid ſanies, perfectly black, and in the higheſt degree offenſive to the ſmell, flowed out. Inflammation, and thickening of the proceſſus vermiformes of the colon, and about ten inches of the ilium, were very viſible.

The

The gall-bladder was much enlarged, and full of very dark-coloured bile. The liver adhered every where to the diaphragm and ſide: the left lobe was much enlarged, extending all the way to the top of the ſpleen, where it alſo adhered ſlightly to the peritonæum of the left ſide. (The ſtate of its ſubſtance, if examined, has not been marked.)

The ſtomach was very much contracted; and the inteſtines, near the mortified portion, were much inflated. There the diameter was rather contracted. A portion of the upper part of the ilium had puſhed through a rent or opening of the omentum, but there was no ſtrangulation of the gut. Nothing further preternatural was obſerved, only there was about an Engliſh pint of greeniſh water in the pelvis.

This appears a complicated caſe. The pathology of it is, however, exceedingly ſimple. A diſeaſed liver was the foundation of the whole. Acrid bile was derived from this ſource; and from the irritation occaſioned by it, and other putreſcent ſordes in the alimentary canal, aroſe inflammation and gangrene of the inteſtines. Could the inflammatory affection of the gut have been moderated, and a little time obtained to draw off the putrid bile and ſordes with which

which the bowels were loaded, there is no ground to doubt the diſeaſe could have been corrected at its origin in the liver, by a mercurial courſe. For this purpoſe, milder and leſs irritating evacuants, perhaps, ought to have been employed; with warm cordials, and perhaps opiates occaſionally, to moderate irritation; and, above all, the early application of a bliſter to the abdomen, where it was ſtrongly indicated by the preſence of topical pain, tenſion, and retraction of the parietes,—appearances that are never equivocal in the abdominal diſorders of India. In this Caſe, alſo, the ſpaſmodic affection ſeems to have ariſen from irritation; occaſioned by topical affection, rather than from diſeaſed bile; and it was but ſlight, and eaſily removed.

THIS variety in the appearances, on diſſection,—topical diſeaſe in the abdominal viſcera evidently connected with it in ſome inſtances, bilious redundancy appearing in others; while in ſome of the worſt and ſevereſt caſes, neither one nor the other could be reaſonably preſumed, created a complete

plete puzzle in all our ſpeculations about the proximate cauſe,—or to what we ought to impute the ſpaſmodic affection, and great irritation on the nervous ſyſtem, which made ſo conſpicuous a part of the diſorder. But about its eſſential character, in all the varieties, as a diſeaſe of extreme debility, we had little doubt. From what cauſe, or how induced, might be difficult to explain, as well as to account for the other phenomena. In whatever way this may be done, or whether we are able to do it ſatisfactorily or not, the thing itſelf is no way different from what I believe will be found a general rule in all caſes of irregularity and overaction in particular portions of the nervous ſyſtem: That they are all but diſeaſes of debility at bottom. Thus epilepſy and hyſteria (where they cannot be traced to a diſtinct irritation) are moſt effectually cured by tonics; and even tetanus itſelf, if we may believe ſome late accounts, has been cured by conſtant libations of wine.

How far the combinations between depraved or redundant ſecretions of bile and the mort de chien might be accidental, or how they might ſtand in the relation of cauſe and effect, antecedent or conſequent, is not eaſy to ſay. We know that certain impreſſions of ſhort and tranſient operation are often followed by remarkable effects upon this and ſome other ſecretions. Thus, ſudden paſſions, or a ſhort over-exerciſe in the heat of the ſun, or lying down to ſleep upon damp graſs after fatiguing exertions, will, in certain ſeaſons, bring on, in our own country, cholera morbus or a bilious fever, even where there were no marks of an increaſed ſecretion of bile previouſly exiſting. We have many examples, again, to ſhew, that certain ſtimuli excite their effects neither on that part of the ſyſtem, to which they are directly applied, nor in proportion to their ordinary force, but according to pre-exiſting tone and pre-diſpoſition. Thus, during the teething period, almoſt every exciting cauſe of diſeaſe produces in children a complaint that ſoon terminates in a bowel-diſorder, and ſo of many others.

Since returning to Europe, I have had occaſion to ſee many caſes of the diſeaſe called in India mort de chien, ſimilar in all reſpects to thoſe we had at Trincomalé, only that they were much milder, and attended with leſs collapſe of the *vires naturæ*. The ſpaſms were exactly of the ſame kind, but confined to the feet, legs and thighs. All of of them happened in the ſummer or autumnal ſeaſon, and none of them proved fatal, except in the caſe of a poor pedlar at Dumfries, for want of proper accommodation and eaſe. One inſtance was in the caſe of Mr J. G., tanner in Edinburgh, whom Dr James Hamilton *primus* was alſo called to ſee.

In all theſe caſes, warm fomentations with cordials were effectual; and the Pil. Opii comp. *Ph. Edin.* were retained on the ſtomach, and anſwered well. No evacuants were made uſe of in any of them. A diſeaſe often to be met with in children during the period of dentition, although it be without cramps, appears to me to partake of the ſame nature with this. It prevails moſt in the ſummer months, and has done ſo more in the courſe of this warm ſummer (1803) than common. They fall into it in the courſe of teething and weaning illneſſes, but often without theſe cauſes being preſent *. The purging with which the diſeaſe commences, becomes frequent and exceſſive; perhaps it is bilious and diſordered at firſt, but at length becomes thin and watery. Conſtant vomitings come on. The feet, legs and hands, are

 very

* See Appendix, No. I.

very apt to become cold. The countenance becomes ſunk, wan, and, if the weather is cold, livid; and the eyes appear hollow, and are ſurrounded with a livid circle. The pulſe is weak, but little altered in frequency. There is the utmoſt degree of flaccidity, relaxation and weakneſs. The child lies in a kind of comatoſe ſtate, with the pupil dilated, and the eyes half-cloſed, and, when rouſed to ſit up, is not able to ſupport the body or head.

Cordials and ſtimulants are in theſe caſes the only remedies that avail any thing. Wine never anſwers this purpoſe with them, but punch does. Bathing the feet and legs in warm water, rubbing them afterwards with warm ſpirits, and wrapping them up in warmed flannel; rubbing brandy or Liniment. anodyn. (Linim. Sapon. cum Opio) warmed, on the ſtomach, and covering it with warmed flannel, and adminiſtering, after every fit of retching, a tea-ſpoonful or two of an adonyne cordial and aſtringent mixture, if long enough perſiſted in, ſeldom fail to remove the complaint. Where we are ſure directions will be properly followed, the better mode will be to adminiſter an opiate daily, or oftener, by glyſter, and to give the cordial and aſtringent mixture the other way. This, however, is ſeldom complied with to our wiſh, and

cannot

cannot be long perfifted in, or perhaps be often enough repeated. Emetics and laxatives, except in the very beginning of the complaint, infallibly do harm.

COPY OF A LETTER, &c.

DEAR SIR, *Fort St George, Feb.* 12. 1774.

I am favoured with yours, and am very happy to hear you have occafioned the army to change its ground; for there can be no doubt, from the circumftances you have mentioned, that their fituation contributes to the frequency and violence of the attacks of this dangerous difeafe, which is, as you have obferved, a true cholera morbus, the fame they had at Trincomalé *.

It is often epidemic among the Blacks, whom it deftroys quickly, as their relaxed habits cannot fupport the effects of fudden evacuations, nor the more powerful operation of difeafed bile.

 In

* This muft refer to fome occafion long anterior to the war of 1782.

In Europe, this difeafe is produced by an increafed acrimony, and increafed fecretion of bile, which operates both ways feverely; but it feldom there brings on fudden weaknefs at the firft onfet. On the contrary, bleeding is often neceffary in the beginning. But when it is epidemic here, it is totally a difeafe of highly putrid bile, which operates on the fyftem as poifon, and brings on fudden proftration of ftrength, and fpafms over the whole furface of the body.

It is a very untractable camp difforder. A warm bed, diluting and blunting medicines, being wanting, and likewife fomentations, &c., and almoft every means to draw the circulation to the furface that are neceffary. However, what can be done under fuch circumftances, fhould be attempted.

In ftrong habits, therefore, when the pulfe keeps up, evacuations fhould be promoted both ways, by a vomit of two or three grains of tartar-emetic to a quart of warm water. After the ftomach feems fufficiently wafhed, a folution of manna and tamarind-water, with Spirit. Nitri dulc. or Cream of Tartar and Manna, largely diluted, fhould be given every half-hour, till it evacuates effectually.

After

After theſe operations, ſaline draughts, in a ſtate of effervеſcence, with Spirit. Lavend., if neceſſary, are material, and ſhould be repeated, like other medicines, as often as they are vomited; warm fomentations of ſalt and water to the belly and legs, and hot bricks to the feet, or a bottle filled with warm water, are very uſeful; and the legs ſhould be rubbed every half hour, to bring on external heat, which enſures the patient, and gives time to complete the cure. In relaxed habits, where the pulſe ſinks ſuddenly, and brings on immediate danger, the ſame method muſt be purſued, but with more caution. The emetics and purges muſt be gentle, and made cordial with wine and Spirit. Lavend. Laudanum muſt be at hand to gain time; and though it is a dangerous expedient to ſuſpend evacuations where putrid bile lurks, yet of two evils the leaſt is to be choſen; for the patient muſt ſink to death in ſuch a caſe, if a reſpite from evacuations, pain and ſpaſms, is not procured. But if a little time can be gained, ſtools can be promoted again. In theſe ſevere caſes, wine and water acidulated, for common drink, will be neceſſary; and ſhould a fever ariſe, purging will remove it. In general, nothing that ruffles is ſafe,

 where

where putrid bile lurks in the habit; and much attention and attendance is required. This diſorder originates in the liver. The ſecretions are diſordered. The bile becomes altered in quality and conſiſtence, and the digeſtion is impaired, until the foundation of ſome illneſs is laid. An accumulation of gelatinous ſtuff in the flexures of the duodenum and colon takes place, which locks up putrid bile, until ſome additional cauſe ſets it in motion. Bleak winds, dews, and inſalutary exhalations, from cold, unventilated, and damp ſituations, give a ſudden check to perſpiration, which proves a ferment to attenuate and ſet in motion this latent miſchief. This is the ſource of the diſeaſe you have in camps, and of all the putrid fluxes and putrid remittents common in the country where hills and woods are. As the diſeaſe often leaves liver-obſtructions behind it, which bring on fluxes, when the men have picked up ſtrength, doſes of rhubarb and calomel will be neceſſary afterwards.

The firſt campaign made in this country, the ſame diſeaſe was horridly fatal to the Blacks; and fifty Europeans of the line were ſeized with it. I have met with many ſingle caſes ſince, and many of of them fatal or dangerous, of different kinds, arifing from putrid bile being difturbed by accidental caufes, or by emetics or purgatives, exhibited before it had been blunted or corrected.

Thefe loofe remarks, in anfwer to yours, I have thrown together, without correctnefs, being hurried at the time with Europe letters. Farewel. I am, Sir, &c. J. PAISLEY.

N. B. I have feen a comatofe difpofition enfue, after the patient has been greatly reduced from the feverity of the fymptoms, and die.

LIVER DISEASES.

HEPATITIS.

EVERY where on the coaft of Coromandel, and, I believe, every where in Lower India, and efpecially in camps, fleets and hofpitals, difeafes of this organ, under one form or other, prevail fo much as to entitle them to be confidered as the grand epidemics of the country.

From the month of July 1782 to March 1783, I believe they conftituted at leaft one-third of our whole

whole hofpital cafes. In the fummer months of 1783, they were ftill more numerous.

When we confider the importance of the organ, and the functions it performs in the fyftem; together with the variety and delicacy of its ftructure, we cannot be furprifed to find it on many occafions, the feat of extenfive and dangerous difeafes. But what the circumftances are that lead to this in India, fo much more than in all other countries under a fimilar latitude, will not be eafily fpecified. All the inflammatory affections of this organ are denominated here, as well as in Europe, by the general name of *Hepatitis*. But *India Hepatitis* includes a variety of affections of this bowel, different in their nature, extent and termination.

From what I obferved in the courfe of attending a very great number of cafes, three different ftates of it were fufficiently diftinguifhable: Hepatitis, with inflammation more or lefs acute: Hepatitis, with chronic inflammation; and Hepatitis with chronic obftruction. The firft runs readily into fuppuration, and at an early period. The fecond only accidentally, or in confequence of neglect, or improper treatment. Both lay the foundation

foundation for long and obftinate fluxes, but are almoft always eafily cured by the proper exhibition of mercury; but now and then terminate in what may be called the third form; a ftate of chronic obftruction. This is always the confequence either of previous inflammation imperfectly removed, or of the healing up of extenfive abfceffes, whether by incifion or otherwife, and is always attended with a coftive belly.

The cafes that terminated fatally with us, were chiefly thofe that were fent on fhore in an advanced ftate of difeafe; and who had, perhaps, been negligently or improperly treated in the beginning. At leaft we attributed to this the great number of patients fent us from the fhips, with large fuppurated livers, during the fummer months of 1783, when we had a large fleet in the country; many of the fhips lately from England, and, of courfe, the furgeons but little acquainted with the India Hepatitis, which differs in many circumftances from that of Europe.

What conftitutes the chief danger and difficulty in managing the complaint, is, that the fymptoms which are primary, and indicate inflammatory affection, are often but very flightly marked;

marked: even where it is in ſuch degree as to run with great readineſs and rapidity into ſuppuration. The pain felt in the ſide is not at all conſtant or acute; the patient himſelf takes little notice of it: ſeldom mentions it unleſs he is aſked about it; and, when you do ſo, he tells you only, he has felt at times ſlight pains about the pit of the ſtomach, or about the right ſide. And it is only from obſerving the ſecondary ſymptoms, ſuch as a flux, or a ſhort dry cough, and pain felt at the top of the ſhoulder, or that there is a degree of fulneſs or tenderneſs on preſſing the region of the liver a little hard, with ſome yellowneſs of the eyes and countenance, that the true ſtate of the diſorder is to be aſcertained.

In about four or five caſes only, out of a great number, the commencement was attended with ſymptoms of pyrexia, *i. e.* heat, thirſt, quickneſs of pulſe and rigors, with an acute pain in the ſide, extending to the top of the ſhoulder. This laſt, which is conſidered in Europe as a conſtant and pathegnomonic ſymptom of the diſeaſe, is far from occurring in every caſe in India. It is not always, when it does occur, in proportion to the degree of fever, or pain of the ſide. It is often felt

felt ſeverely when the laſt is but inconſiderable, and ſometimes continues long after it is gone off; or it frequently remains during the whole time the liver is in a ſtate of ulceration, or of much obſtruction.

Whether it be a more conſtant attendant on the membranous or parenchymatous inflammation, I was unable to determine. But in ſeveral caſes that ended in large and deep-ſeated ulcerations, it never took place: while it was common in others that were only ſlight, and eaſily removed.

Whenever it did occur, it ſerved to render the nature of the diſeaſe very certain. It is moſt diſtinctly felt at the very point of the ſhoulder, rather behind; and is aggravated on moving the arm. In ſome caſes, where the left lobe of the liver was known to be affected, the ſame thing was felt at the top of the left ſhoulder. And in one caſe, the patient complained of a ſimilar pain in both.

Though the diſeaſe commences often without much pain, heat, or quickneſs of pulſe; yet this is not univerſal; for ſometimes there is both quickneſs and fulneſs in the pulſe; and in two caſes there were conſiderable rigors: but moſt commonly

monly theſe leading circumſtances were wanting. We only found that the patient had had a flux, which had laſted for ſome time, with more or leſs ſtraining and griping; and perhaps paſſed ſome blood with his ſtools, which were ſlimy and bilious; and that this flux had reſiſted the common remedies, or had been but little relieved by repeated evacuants. And when we came to examine him about the ſtate of his liver, he would ſay he had at times felt pain in his right ſide. And on examining the part, a fulneſs could perhaps be obſerved under the ends of the falſe ribs, towards the pit of the ſtomach; and that he complained of ſome pain upon preſſing the part a little hard, or upon taking in a full inſpiration. By theſe ſymptoms, the nature of the complaint was rendered fully certain, though he had formerly obſerved no pain there, or had but little or no fever, nor ever felt any pain in the ſhoulder; eſpecially if to theſe were added a ſallow look, and yellowiſh caſt of the tunica albuginea, which never fail in ſome degree to attend every liver affection in this country. The flux very often precedes every other ſymptom of the inflammation, and is the moſt conſtant attendant upon it: except in a few caſes where the attack

tack is more fudden and accute, and then a fhort dry tickling cough is often prefent. Both are fymptoms only, and are cured along with the inflammation itfelf, and by the fame means.

In fome cafes the flux remains long, and proves obftinate; moft probably in confequence of topical affection of fome part of the inteftine, occafioned by the irritation of difeafed and acrid fecretions. This appears evident in the advanced ftate of liver-fluxes, by the bloody ftools and griping felt in the lower part of the abdomen. Fluxes, we found to be fo conftant attendants in this country upon a difeafed ftate of the liver, that after a little experience, whenever they refifted even for a fhort time the ordinary methods of cure, we became immediately fufpicious of the ftate of that organ,—that it was affected either with inflammation, or ulcerated, or in a ftate of inflammatory obftruction. We knew from diffection that obftructed mefentery had alfo fometimes a concern; efpecially in thofe cafes that were of long ftanding, and attended with relaxed habit, and a debilitated ftate of the organs of digeftion: Such patients are here called *Lienterics*. We had at all times a great number of cafes that were fimple, arifing from

from a ſuperabundant or diſordered ſtate of the bilious ſecretion; and we had ſome occaſionally from irregularities, and from cold and obſtructed perſpiration. But we found ſo often affections of the liver at the bottom of the complaint, or appearing in the courſe of it, as to make us cautious and diſtruſtful in almoſt every caſe. True dyſentery never appeared in the hoſpital; nor do I believe it is ever to be met with in Lower India: at leaſt without being imported thither. We had enough of fluxes from diſeaſed bile; with highly putrid and dyſenteric ſymptoms as the diſeaſe proceeded in its courſe: but theſe were of a nature totally different from true dyſentery, and began in a different quarter,—in the upper part of the inteſtinal canal.

In ſome caſes, after all the ſymptoms of inflammation in the liver had been removed, and the patient had been reſtored to his former ſtate of health, appetite and ſtrength, and a clear countenance, ſlight pains of the ſide would continue to be felt at times, and a hardneſs of the bowel could be perceived; but I never ſaw any very remarkable enlargement of it—Large Scirrhous Liver, or, what is called, *Liver-grown.*

While

While this ſtate of hardneſs and pain continued, it was eaſily aggravated by any irregularity ; particularly in drinking, and it was always attended with a coſtive belly ; ſo that it was difficult to get any thing to purge the patients freely, except caſtor oil. The ſame thing was obſervable in ſeveral caſes where abſceſſes of the liver had been cut for and healed up. But there were not many inſtances of relapſe in the hoſpital, where the diſeaſe returned again, or advanced to the ſtate of ulceration, (though ſome pain might remain at times), after the patients had gone through a proper courſe of mercury.

The period of the diſeaſe was of no certain extent or duration. If the acceſſion was with pyrexia, or acute ſymptoms, the progreſs was more rapid than where it was ſlower, and where theſe were wanting. If it was neglected, or wrong treated in the beginning, it ſometimes ran very ſuddenly into ſuppuration, even where there were no acute ſymptoms. Perſons who had been long in the country, and lived irregular, were more ſubject to it than the more temperate.

Occaſional cauſes were not very diſtinguiſhable ; but I ſometimes imagined, that long-ſtanding bilious fluxes had the effect of inducing diseafe in the liver itself; for certain appearances of this sometimes took place in cases of such fluxes so long after they had come on, and where nothing of the kink was observable at first, as could not have subsisted where we were so much on our guard against this affection. The disease in the organ is, perhaps, excited by the acrimony of its own secretion.

When the inflammation was not soon resolved by the exhibition of mercury, the substance of the liver ran speedily into a state of suppuration. An abscess formed, too often of very large extent. A great deal of the substance of the liver came to be broken down and destroyed; the matter sometimes finding its way by the gall-ducts, which soon brings on a putrid flux, and destroys the patient. When the abscess was on the convex part of the liver, the matter not unfrequently made its way through the diaphragm, eroded the lungs, and came to be spit up. In two cases of this sort, where the ulcer had extended deep, and eroded the gall-ducts, much bile was brought up by coughing mixed with sanious matter, plainly distinguishable, not only by the colour, but the bitterness of

taste.

tafte. One patient was opened after death, and we found the paffage through the diaphragm not larger than would allow a very fmall quill to pafs. The liver was a mafs of ulcerations and putrid matter, and almoft the whole of the right lung was obliterated; the fpace filled up with a fpongy loofe membranous fubftance, difpofed in thin layers. What remained of the lung was fhrivelled up to the top of the thorax, and very knotty and hard. There muft be very few inftances of fuppurations of the liver healing up in this way. We had feven or eight of thefe cafes at the hofpital, but all of them proved fatal.

When the abfcefs forms on the fore part of the liver, and is not feated very deep in its fubftance, the matter frequently points outwards, forming an indiftinct kind of tumour; which appears ofteneft juft under the ends of the firft falfe ribs, or between them and the pit of the ftomach; fometimes right over it; and one was opened near to the ends of the falfe ribs on the left fide. In other cafes, the tumour forms more backwards within the ribs. One was opened between the fourth and fifth falfe ribs.

This tumour ſometimes appears ſuddenly, and, when the ulcer is not deep-ſeated, is tolerably circumſcribed and prominent. But unfortunately the ſeat of the matter, in many inſtances, is not exactly pointed out by ſuch a tumour at all. There is only a fulneſs and hardneſs, or rather a general ſwelling, which pits a little on preſſing it with the points of the fingers: or, before any external tumour is formed, by which the ſeat of the matter can be exactly known, it has ſpread too far below; has formed a large abſceſs within the ſubſtance of the liver; and, when at laſt an inciſion is made, and the matter is let out, it has ſpread and deſtroyed much of the ſubſtance of the organ; or it has found, or afterwards finds its way by the gall-ducts, and brings on a fatal putrid flux. The ulcer does not fill up and heal; the matter furniſhed becomes acrid and ſtinking, and produces new inflammation, and ſpreading ulcerations. This was the unfortunate courſe of a great many caſes we had in the year 1782. Out of ten patients in which the abſceſſes were opened, we only ſaved two. In one of them, the tumour was diſtinguiſhable the firſt time he complained of any pain in his ſide; and he never felt any in the

ſhoulder.

ſhoulder. He was in the hoſpital for the cure of an ulcer, and only had a ſlight flux for ſix or eight days; for which ſome evacuating medicines had been given him. The tumour in two days was prominent enough to be opened. The ulcer in the liver was of no great extent, and the matter was white, and without any bad ſmell. The other had complained longer, but the tumour was not at all elevated nor circumſcribed. An inciſion was, however, made near an inch into the ſubſtance of the liver; but no matter being come at, and a conſiderable hæmorrhage enſuing, it was thought unſafe to proceed farther. The matter, in two or three days, made its way to the opening. It was in no great quantity, and the patient ſoon got well upon a mercurial courſe *.

* A ſimilar inſtance came under my care at Dumfries, in the year 1785. A boy about eleven years of age, had evident ſymptoms of inflamed liver, and of ſuppuration having taken place within the falſe ribs, pretty far back, where they were evidently puſhed out and elevated; forming at one place a kind of indiſtinct tumour. With ſome difficulty I perſuaded the boy himſelf, and his parents, to ſubmit to have an opening made at this place; and proceeded ſo far as to cut through the ſkin, and divide the intercoſtal muſcle, meaning to

In the ſummer months of 1783, ſtill a greater number underwent this operation, and only three or four were recovered by it.

There never was any danger in making the inciſion. The nature of the complaint had always become clear enough before any thing of this kind was reſolved on; and if there was any thing of a tumour at all, we were ſure that, previous to the formation of this, the inflammation had produced adheſion between the membrane of the liver and peritoneum, ſo as to exclude all the contiguous organs from coming in the way of the knife. I never ſaw either the ſtomach or colon, the only organs that could poſſibly interfere, affected by the inflammation, or that the matter had made its way into either of them. In ſeveral large ſuppurations of the liver, we ſometimes found

---

to puſh a lancet into the tumour; but the boy himſelf got frightened, as well as the people about him, and would ſubmit to nothing farther. In the courſe of a week, however, matter in conſiderable quantity began to appear; but the opening being by this time contracted, it inſinuated itſelf ſeveral ways under the ſkin, and formed ſeveral new openings for itſelf; whereby, in the courſe of ſome time, the diſeaſe of his liver was completely removed, and the openings all healed up.

found the dreſſings tinged with bile, but never any appearance that a communication had been formed with the colon or ſtomach; even where the patient ſurvived the opening a long time, and the diſeaſe proved fatal at laſt.

The external inciſion was generally made near to and parallel with the ends of the ribs, and this was ſometimes undertaken, and the matter found where no diſtinct fluctuation could be felt. Caution was always obſerved in making it; to proceed ſlowly, to wipe away the blood, and examine the parts before every ſtroke of the ſcalpel, until the matter was found. It was neceſſary to carry the inciſion of the teguments much farther than was required for giving vent to the diſcharge, as the opening was very ready to cloſe up, unleſs kept open by tents, which were hurtful, by confining the matter, and cauſing it to ſpread within. Of whatever kind this was, it very ſoon became exceedingly acrid and ſtinking, ſoon after it was expoſed to the acceſs of the air. Generally it was ſo at the very firſt diſcharge; commonly of a thick greaſy conſiſtence, of a liver-colour, full of red lumps ſwimming in it, and of a peculiar ſmell. This we thought the worſt kind, as

 none

none recovered where it was of this appearance. In others, it was more thin and pale-coloured, but equally acrid and ill-ſmelled. All of it tinged the probe with a brown colour. Seldom, indeed, was there any thing like good pus. In one caſe it was a clear fluid, reſembling the water of an hydatid.

It was common to throw in injections, with Mel Roſ. or Tincture of Myrrh, three times a-day, and to give bark. In only one caſe did the bark ſeem to produce any favourable change in the condition of the matter. In all the reſt, it did no manner of good. In by far the greateſt number, the ulcers were of very great extent. Two, three, or even more pounds of matter, were ſometimes diſcharged at the firſt opening; and often the finger could be turned all round within it, without reaching any part of the ſubſtance of the liver. Where there was ſo great a deſtruction of ſubſtance, the proſpect of recovery could be but very ſmall.

Cure.—Whenever the diſeaſe came on with a conſiderable degree of fever, with acute and conſtant pain in the ſide and ſhoulder, ſome bleeding was practiſed: but in other caſes it was never done;

done; and indeed to the extent to which it could well be carried in a warm climate, and in relaxed habits, it ſeldom procured much relief. A large bliſter, applied over the part affected, had much better effects. Oftener than once it appeared to have removed the inflammation entirely. When it was intended to follow the mercurial courſe by frictions upon the ſide, this came to be in the way of that; but was never without effect in relieving the pain of the ſide and ſhoulder; and cough, when theſe were preſent. Whether bleeding or bliſtering were employed, it was always of conſequence to clear the bowels, and carry down the diſeaſed ſecretions, by a purgative or two; ſalts and manna, in gentle doſes, or Decoct. Tamarind. cum Sen.; or if a ſtronger was wanted, caſtor oil. Sometimes a few cooling powders, compoſed of nitre, gum-arabic and Cream of Tartar, were given for a few days at firſt, along with the mercurial frictions; eſpecially where there was heat, thirſt and pyrexia, with a view to abate theſe, and render the operation of the mercury milder. Some thought this rendered the exhibition of it more ſucceſsful and ſafer; and I have obſerved relief obtained from the uſe of theſe before the mercu-

ry-

ry could have entered the fyftem in fuch quantity as to produce it.

In all other circumftances, or as foon as the pain of the fide, heat and fever, had been a little abated by the ufe of thefe remedies, mercury was immediately had recourfe to, and the courfe pufhed on, as quickly as poffible, without any regard to the ftate of the bowels, even where there was a conftant flux, with bloody ftools and tenefmus; fometimes where even a good deal of heat, thirft and general fever were prefent, provided the pulfe was not hard, and the pain of the fide had fomewhat abated, or was not very conftant and acute. Our dependance upon it was fo great, unlefs where it was fuppofed the diforder had already advanced to fuppuration, that the more preffing the fymptoms feemed to be, we were the more anxious, with the precautions already mentioned, to get the fyftem fpeedily and fully charged with it. Its good effect in every fpecies of liver difeafe, except in the ftate of ulceration and fimple diforder of its fecretion, viz. fimple bilious fever and flux, were fo apparent, that we had recourfe to it with the fame confidence as in lues venerea. Scarcely was it ever obferved to increafe the heat

and

and fever, or to aggravate the pain of the ſide or cough; and the bowel diſorder, flux and bloody ſtools, were often removed by it alone, or they diſappeared under its uſe without any other remedies; ſo that I began ſometimes to ſuſpect that our precautions and apprehenſions about its aggravating effects in certain circumſtances of the diſeaſe, had been imaginary only.

A flux is ſo conſtant an attendant upon inflammation and inflammatory obſtruction of the liver, or obſtructed meſentery, that very often, when it proved obſtinate, we had recourſe to mercury for its removal, when we had no other foundation for ſuſpecting an unſound condition of theſe organs than merely the flux itſelf; and generally, if the conſtitution was ſound, with perfect ſucceſs. Often, while we were going on with our mercurial courſes for the cure of inflamed liver, and ſuppoſed it to be nearly, or fully removed, a return of the flux would take place on our abating the mercury, and we were obliged to puſh it on again, and continue it longer, for the removal of this ſymptom, after all pain of the ſide had been long removed.

The

The preparations of mercury moſt generally uſed, were a pill compoſed of a grain and a half of calomel, and two of rhubarb and ſoap. Of theſe, two were given every night and morning, and if it was thought neceſſary to have the mouth ſoon affected, a drachm of mercurial ointment was alſo rubbed in along the ſide every night. The blue pill was ſometimes uſed in place of the calomel, and anſwered equally well, eſpecially where it was wiſhed the mouth ſhould be ſoon affected, and the bowel diſorder was not great; but where this was the caſe, I was certain the rhubarb and calomel pills ſooner corrected it. It may be thought, much of the mercury would run off and be loſt in this way, but this did not appear; for the mouth became as ſoon affected with either of theſe, as by the mode of friction. This, however, is not ſo eaſily excited in India, and goes ſooner off than in colder climates. After the mouth became ſore, the mercury was continued in ſmaller doſes for two or three weeks, or until every ſymptom of the diſeaſe had diſappeared; and we had reaſon to ſuppoſe the inflammation quite removed, and the liver reſtored to a natural healthy ſtate; not merely till the pain of the ſide was removed, and the

bowel

bowel diforder had been fully corrected, but till the patient recovered his natural appetite and ftrength, and the fallownefs and yellow colour of the countenance was exchanged for the clear look of returning health. Few other medicines were, in general, neceffary during the ufe of the mercury; except now and then fome eafy laxatives, fuch as fmall dofes of Rhubarb and ipecacuanha; or Rhubarb and Cream of Tartar, when the other was not fufficiently active to carry off the irritating matters; or emollient glyfters to remove tenefmus.

Such is the hiftory of the acute ftate of liver inflammation as it appeared with us; and fuch was the general mode of treatment. Where the circumftances were tolerably favourable, we fucceeded, in almoft every inftance, in curing it. But very often the patients were too far gone before they came under our care. The difeafe had run on to a ftate of fuppuration, or was too far in progrefs towards it, before mercury could be introduced to check and prevent it. Whether ulcerations of any confiderable fize were healed up by it, I could not be very certain. But from what we faw on diffection, in fome cafes where the patient died afterwards of other complaints, and had

been

been under difeafe of this organ, I was pretty certain, that fmall ulcers on the external furface had been healed up under its ufe. (See the cafe of John Holland.)

Befides the acute, there was another inflammatory affection of the liver, of a more chronic nature, which laid the foundation for fluxes of a more obftinate and intractable kind than thofe we have mentioned: Or, we had a number of fluxes, attended with griping and ftraining at the beginning, but which in the end became mere lienteric diarrhœas, without being attended with either; until the laft ftages, when the rectum came to be affected by the conftant depofition of acrid bile and undigefted aliments, and then pain and tenefmus became again very troublefome. In thefe kind of fluxes, the liver always felt tender to the touch; but the affection feemed to be different from the acute inflammation, and did not run fo readily into a ftate of fuppuration, except through neglect, wrong treatment, or great irregularity. Obftructions of the mefentery appeared, in feveral inftances, to have occafioned fluxes of a fimiliar nature and obftinacy. We were certain of this in three different patients that were opened

opened after death. The liver was found to be in a ſound ſtate; but the meſentery was thickened, and full of hard knotty enlarged glands, ſome of them of conſiderable ſize, with its veſſels enlarged and turgid: the coats of the inteſtines alſo, in many places, thickened and contracted.

In theſe, as well as in thoſe that depended on acute inflammation of the liver, it was a common thing for the patients to paſs blood with their ſtools, ſometimes in conſiderable quantities. But I conſtantly obſerved, where it was not merely the effect of ſtraining, it was paſſed pure and unmixed; and was moſt probably the conſequence of congeſtion, and rupture of ſome ſmall blood-veſſel low down in the canal. In other caſes, ariſing from chronic inflammation, the ſtools were much tinged with green, or a green mixed with a yellow colour, or of a dark-red approaching to a black; and whenever they continued long of this appearance, and the patient had a ſallow look, and yellowneſs of the albuginea, even although there were no ſymptoms of acute inflammation of the liver preſent, no ſort of benefit was derived from any courſe of medicines that were only palliative or corrective. And if we had no ſucceſs by mercurial

curial alteratives, pushed perhaps beyond that degree so as to affect the mouth for a while at first, and continued for some time in gentler doses, we infallibly lost our patient. The flux became more and more frequent; brought on a total relaxation of the intestines; and the functions of digestion became totally lost; every thing they took ran through them, in an undigested state; a slow fever and wasting came on, which in the end proved fatal.

Where the constitution had not been much impaired, the bloody stools and bilious sordes began to disappear on the use of mercury; the patient regained some appetite and strength, which enabled him to bear the operation of the medicine, until health was gradually restored by it. But in the beginning occasional laxatives behoved to be joined with it, for keeping the intestines clear of accumulation of diseased secretions, more than in the case of acute inflammation.

For restoring the tone of the stomach and intestines, light infusions of bitters, the Margosa leaf and Elix. Vitriol. were employed. But bark and astringents were cautiously avoided.

There

There was a ſtate of obſtruction in the liver, which ſometimes ſucceeded both the acute inflammation and the cure of thoſe ulcers that had been healed up after inciſion. Coſtiveneſs in theſe caſes, was always troubleſome. Caſtor oil was the moſt effectual in overcoming this. When pain became conſiderable, if the patient had tolerable ſtrength of conſtitution, the repetition of a mercurial courſe, in ſeveral inſtances, removed this entirely. Bliſters over the part, gave temporary relief; and a ſeton over the region of the liver, was found, in ſome inſtances, of great benefit.

CASE.

The following caſe, which occurred on board the Seahorſe ſoon after my arrival in the country, and which was recorded on the event, well deſerves to be hung up *in terrorem* againſt the attacks of this inſidious diſeaſe, and pointedly ſhews the danger of being miſled, by attending to ſymptoms that are but ſecondary, while we overlook thoſe that, though they may be more ſlightly marked, are primary and pathognomic.

William Quail, ſeaman on board the Seahorſe, on the 6th of June 1782, complained of ſlight flux, without much ſtraining or gripes. Having been on ſhore for the cure of a ſcorbutic ulcer, his complaint was imputed to ſome irregularity; to drinking too much of the cocoa-nut juice, called *toady*, or too free a uſe of vegetables; and a ſlight purge or two were only preſcribed for him. On the 9th he was ſuddenly ſeized with a cold ſhivering fit, which was ſevere, and followed by heat and ſweating. This was repeated four times in forty-eight hours, but the periods were not perfectly exact. During the fit, his pulſe was quick, and his ſkin was hot; even when he was under the rigours. In the intervals, he was free from fever, and in all reſpects pretty well. He ſaid he had felt at times pain in his right ſide, but it was not conſtant or ſevere. He mentioned alſo his right ſhoulder, which, though I had then never ſeen hepatitis, ſuggeſted a ſuſpicion of his liver being affected, and I knew that it was a frequent diſeaſe in India; but he mentioned alſo that he had a pain acroſs his loins, and, at times, felt pain in the left ſhoulder; and ſuppoſing that hepatitis was always to be diſtinguiſhed by acute and conſtant pain in the ſide

and

and ſhoulder, with a conſtant ſtate of fever, and the fits, though ſomewhat irregular, reſembling thoſe of intermittents, the idea of hepatitis was given up, and the complaint was ſuppoſed to be of the *aguiſh* kind, ariſing from ſome foulneſs in the *primæ viæ*. He had an emetic and laxative, and, after the ſecond fit was over, bark in pretty large doſes. This was continued for two days. The fits went off, but he had more fever. On the 13th he again mentioned pain of his ſide, and that his flux, which had been relieved, was returned. It was now intended to put him on a courſe of mercury, and, preparatory to this, his ſide was fomented and a bliſter applied over it; which removed the pain entirely. He had nitrous powders in his drink, a doſe of ſoluble tartar, and ſome ſmall doſes of rhubarb and ipecacuanha to the 17th, when he complained of a fulneſs and oppreſſion at his ſtomach. On inſpection, there was no appearance of ſwelling, but it was painful on being preſſed. A ſmall doſe of tartar emetic was given him, which evacuated him downwards. On the 20th, he complained of oppreſſion of breathing, and began to cough. The emetic tartar was repeated *ad vomitum*. Next day he began to ſpit up bloody ſtuff with his cough. This ſoon changed into pure pus, and in a ſhort time to pure bile, which continued to the 25th, when he died. He paſſed alſo yellow purulent-like matter downwards, in conſiderable quantity. After the bliſter, he never complained of any pain of his ſide or ſhoulder, but at the pit of his ſtomach. And the true nature of his diſeaſe was not fully underſtood till it ſhewed itſelf too plainly, and too late, by the ſpitting of bile.

The liver had been inflamed from the beginning, and the diſeaſed ſtate of this organ had been at the bottom of the flux and fits of pyrexiæ; yet all this while the pain of the ſide and ſhoulder were but ſlight, never conſtant, and were eaſily removed. But there is not the leaſt doubt, if he had been narrowly queſtioned, a degree of pain in the region of the liver, would have been found to exiſt from the very firſt acceſſion of the flux, though he had attended but little to it himſelf; or, at leaſt, he would have been ſenſible of ſome ſoreneſs or tenderneſs to the touch, on preſſing the part a little hard, or in making a full inſpiration, or ſome fulneſs at leaſt would have been diſcovered; and the early exhibition of mercury would, in all probability, have ſucceeded in ſaving him.

This

This was an inſtructive caſe, although at the poor man's expence. More experience, acquired in a ſhort time, removed all riſk of ſimilar blunders, and rendered the diagnoſis in ſuch caſes much more eaſy and certain.

BILIOUS DISEASES.

BILIOUS FEVER AND FLUX.

By this title is not to be underſtood any determinate ſpecies of fever neceſſarily connected with a bowel diſorder, as in dyſentery; or any ſpecies of idiopathic diſeaſe of the febrile kind whatever. The fever, on the contrary, is purely and perfectly ſymptomatic; and I am indeed doubtful, whether, on the coaſt of India, there be any other. Typhus, ſynochus or ſynocha, ſcarlatina and eryſipelas, were unknown to us; and both remittents and intermittents appeared only at the hoſpital as ſymptomatics, depending on diſordered and ſuperabundant bile, and other vitiated accumulations in the firſt paſſages.

But, although the fever makes no neceſſary or eſſential part of the diſeaſe, it is ſeldom entirely wanting where the bowel-diſorder has been of any ſtanding; and the ſymptoms of it often run ſo high, as to create no ſmall additional danger, and render the management of it a matter of much delicacy: So that it becomes highly neceſſary to have a particular eye to it, both in the deſcription and treatment of the complaint.

This kind of fever and flux was not attended with more yellowneſs of the ſkin, eyes, or urine, than commonly accompanies all the India diſeaſes where the liver or its ſecretion are concerned. The flux frequently precedes the acceſſion of fever, or the latter only appears occaſionally or tranſiently, according to the degree of acrimony and accumulation of diſordered ſecretions in the ſtomach and upper part of the inteſtinal canal; and its exacerbations and alleviations follow pretty exactly the degree of theſe. The fever never remains a day after the bowel-diſorder is fully corrected, but for the moſt part terminates ſooner, or is only occaſionally renewed and lighted up by the renewal of freſh accumulations.

That

That both flux and fever are produced and maintained by a ſuperabundant and vitiated condition of the bilious ſecretion, in the firſt inſtance, is abundantly plain from the nature of the diſcharges, and the diſorder induced on the alvine functions.

In relation to the ſtomach, it is evinced by nauſea and ſickneſs, bitter taſte in the mouth, loaded yellow tongue, and want of appetite.

In the upper part of the inteſtinal canal, it is ſhewn by anxiety, ſenſe of weight, and fulneſs about the præcordia, pain, tumour and fulneſs, with ſome ſoreneſs and tenderneſs on preſſing the part with the fingers.

In the middle portion of the tract, it is evident by the tumid abdomen, with tenderneſs and uneaſineſs on preſſure, gripes, flatus, borborygmi, ſpaſmodic and ſhifting pains; and that uneaſy ſenſation which may be called *bowel-ſickneſs*; diſtinguiſhable from ſtomach affection, as conſiſting in that ſenſation that ariſes in cholic, or whenever acrimonious or irritating matters are put into motion in the inteſtines by the action of their coats, whether from the addition of a purgative ſtimulus or otherwiſe.

In the lower portion of the inteſtinal canal, eſpecially in the rectum, and particularly in the latter ſtages of the diſeaſe, it is teſtified by griping, ſtraining, teneſmus, mucous, and bloody ſtools, of a deep bilious, or of a ſanious or putrid appearance. More or leſs of the ſame appearances are to be found in the diſcharges by ſtool in every ſtage of the complaint. But unleſs where topical affection has early taken place, the firſt diſcharges conſiſt more of ſlime and bilious matters, and in larger quantity, than in the ſubſequent periods.

The cauſe from which the diſeaſe had its origin, always appeared to be ſuperabundance and acrimony of bile, inducing diſorder in the ſtomach, and in the ſecretions of the upper part of the canal. But the diſorder was not long confined to this portion, but made its way downwards by degrees, whereby it had the appearance of being divided into different ſtages; which, however, had no other diſtinction, nor any certain periods of duration.

The occaſional or exciting cauſes were, in general; irregularity in living, great exertion and fatigue under expoſure to the heat of the ſun. Of this we had frequent experience among our con-

valeſcents

valefcents who were allowed to walk out of the hofpital: and in the number of patients received from the fhips, parties employed in watering, and other duties on fhore. In moft of thefe, the attack was fudden and fevere, and attended with a high degree of fever. The pulfe fometimes hard, but always very frequent; tongue and fkin dry, hot and parched; and the patient very foon became delirious. By far the greater number were fent us from the fhips with the difeafe in a more advanced ftate; with the tongue thickly covered with a yellow cruft; with a fmall and quick pulfe, pale funk or fallow countenance; great heat, pain, tenfion and tumour of the abdomen; ftupor and infenfibility; now and then with wild phrenfy and delirium; and fometimes with cold extremities, hiccup, and cold fweats.

In this ftate, it is hardly neceffary to fay, they generally died. Inflammation and gangrene of the inteftines foon came on. The mildeft evacuants were either rejected from the ftomach, or before it could be brought to bear fuch as could be any way effectual, the difeafe had made too great progrefs to be arrefted by any remedies; or the mildeft laxations we could employ, brought on fo much irritation as greatly exafperated all the

fymptoms;

ſymptoms; and cordials, diluents, fomentations and glyſters, were ſometimes all we had to truſt to.

In many inſtances among thoſe taken ill at the hoſpital, the acceſſion of the diſeaſe was obſerved to be much more gradual; and it ſometimes affected thoſe of the moſt careful and regular modes of life.

A purging, with more or leſs griping and ſtraining, would begin to come on, attended with an uneaſy ſenſation of weight about the præcordia; anxiety, depreſſion and lowneſs of ſpirits, with ſtools of a bilious colour, a dark-yellow, with a mixture of green; and this would continue ſometimes for weeks, the patient all the while going about, and enjoying a tolerable ſtate of appetite and health; till at laſt the bilious ſecretion came to be ſo increaſed and vitiated, as to diſorder all the functions of the ſtomach and bowels, and to bring on fever, with an amazing redundancy of bile, which would often continue long after the fever was removed. In moſt caſes, the degree of fever was pretty much in proportion to the cumulation in the upper part of the alimentary canal, and kept pace pretty exactly with the ſtate of evacuation

cuation made from it; ſometimes diſappearing in a ſhort time, or being only renewed at intervals in the progreſs of the complaint, or when new accumulations had taken place.

In this, which might be called the *Firſt Stage* of the diſorder, there was generally more or leſs fulneſs at the pit of the ſtomach, with ſome ſoreneſs or tenderneſs on preſſure there, or rather between the pit of the ſtomach and right hypochondrium; or between it and the umbilicus, towards the right ſide. And ſo much ſuſpicion and anxiety being neceſſarily attached to the ſtate of the liver in every India flux, much perplexity was apt to ariſe from this feeling in ſimple bilious diſorders. But in general the true index was to be found in attending to the circumſtances of the caſe, and the concomitant ſymptoms.

The pain here was more dull, deep-ſeated, and lower down, farther from the ends of the ribs than where the liver was concerned; and where the fever and bowel irritation was not ſo great, as to prevent a briſk purgative from being given, ſo as to carry down a load of diſeaſed congeſtions from the turns of the duodenum, the pain and uneaſineſs

uneaſineſs in this caſe will be greatly relieved by it. But no ſuch relief is obtained from them in hepatic affection.

Pretty acute pains are alſo ſometimes felt in the courſe of the diſeaſe in various places of the abdomen. Some portion of the inteſtine becomes affected with pain of the ſpaſmodic kind; perhaps with ſtricture and accumulation of the contents: and this not unfrequently happens in ſome part of the arch of the colon. In one caſe, where a pain of this kind kept pretty much fixed about the edge of the liver, much ſuſpicion was occaſioned by it about the ſtate of that organ: but from obſerving, that it alternated with ſimilar pains in other places of the abdomen, and from the relief obtained by purgatives, or from the motion through the inteſtines being free, the true nature of the caſe was aſcertained; and fully confirmed in the event, by the complete recovery of the patient, without any one remedy for the cure of liver-diſeaſe being employed.

Another ſymptom, often attendant upon the febrile ſtate of this diſeaſe, and indeed very commonly felt by ſome perſons in India, whenever bile predominates in the firſt paſſages, is a torpor or numbneſs

numbneſs in ſome of the limbs, ariſing in ſome caſes to a degree of paralyſis. The right arm is often affected in this way; ſometimes only the outſide of the hand, or two or three of the outer fingers are only affected. Others have ſpaſms and cramps in the legs or feet.

The horridly-fatal diſeaſe, commonly known, when I was in India, by the name of the *Mort de Chien*, which has been already deſcribed, was conſidered by ſome of the firſt practitioners there, as entirely a diſeaſe of putrid bile. Though I did not at all embrace this opinion, but conſidered the two diſorders as ſpecific and diſtinct in their nature, though frequently in accidental or occaſional combination; yet both at Trincomalé, when we had the diſeaſe in the Seahorſe, and in the ſummer months of the year 1783, while it was frequent in the fleet, we had patients ſent to the hoſpital from the ſhips, under bilious fever and flux, affected with the ſame ſort of external ſpaſms and cramps as take place in that diſorder. But then, in all theſe caſes, the ſpaſms were much milder; the diſeaſe much more tractable; the ſpaſms appeared to be only ſecondary; and the exiſtence of bilious plethora was perfectly conſpicuous.

The

The ſame ſpaſmodic affection occurred alſo in ſome inſtances among our people at the hoſpital in the courſe of bilious and liver fluxes of ſome ſtanding.

In the firſt ſtage of bilious fever and flux, along with ſome pain, tumour, and fulneſs of the abdomen, with preternatural heat of the part, and ſoreneſs on preſſure; the tongue was dry and yellow, and the eyes and urine had ſome tinge of the ſame colour. The latter ſometimes tinged the linen with a duſky brown or yellow; but this was very unſteady and variable.

Very often there was little purging or griping when the patient lay ſtill in bed, or while the contents of the bowels were not diſturbed, and put into motion by laxatives; but as ſoon as their action was excited by this means, violent pain and griping were produced, with a conſtant redundancy of bile and diſordered ſecretions, which often continued for an indefinite period; and if theſe were not as conſtantly carried forward by promoting the action of the whole inteſtinal canal, a return, or aggravation of the fever, and all the ſymptoms, was the infallible conſequence.

The

The ſtate of the abdomen was a pretty ſure index of the quantity and degree of theſe accumulations; but this was by no means to be taken from the patient's own deſcription or feelings, but from the degree of fulneſs and tenderneſs on preſſure; from the effect the firſt exhibition of purgatives or glyſters had in exciting pain, griping and ſickneſs; or from the appearance of the diſcharge produced by them. This indeed was varied at different periods of the diſorder. Conſtantly there was a greeniſh colour, varying from a dun and duſky yellow, to a dark and dirty black. The laſt predominates during the febrile period. I have ſeen them, for weeks, of the colour of moſs-water. Sometimes there was more of a red colour, like chocolate or coffee grounds; and when this was the caſe, with much pain, tumour, and tenſion of the abdomen, the diſeaſe often ended in topical inflammation and gangrene of the inteſtines.

When the ſtomach and upper part of the inteſtinal canal had been pretty well cleared, and the diſeaſed ſecretions carried downwards by repeated evacuations, what may be called the *Second Stage* of the diſorder commenced. Partial accumulations

tions of diſeaſed matters ſtill continued to be renewed from time to time ; and the diſorder ſettled lower and lower down, accompanied with much griping and ſtraining to ſtool ; often with ſome blood in the ſtools, and frequently with ſome degree of dyſuria,—pain and difficulty of voiding urine ; but with intervals, and a conſiderable abatement of fever, pain and general diſorder of the abdomen: or, inſtead of being tumid, the abdomen rather became ſhrunk and retracted, with the ſkin tenſe, dry and hot, and the pain more confined to a particular ſpot, indicating more of topical affection ; which we found on diſſection to have affected in ſeveral inſtances the ſigmoid flexure of the colon, and upper part of the rectum.

Irregular ſpaſmodic contractions of the lower bowels, eſpecially of the rectum, frequently took place ; preventing the free and regular propulſion of the contents of the inteſtines ; and rendered the frequent exhibition of glyſters and purgatives neceſſary, even though the ſtools were perfectly liquid, and in large quantity, whenever the mildeſt of theſe were given.

If

If the diſeaſe continued long in this ſtate, eſpecially if the patient was of a reduced habit, or much debilitated by long reſidence in the country, it ended in what was conſidered as its *Third* and *Laſt Stage*,—a lienteric or colliquative diarrhœa. This was often of long ſtanding, and terminated fatally, long after fever and redundancy of bile had entirely diſappeared. The patients continued to be haraſſed with frequent watery and liquid or mucous ſtools; whatever they took by the mouth paſſed through them in a half-digeſted ſtate, till a kind of low hectic, and waſting maraſmus, concluded the ſcene.

In this ſtate of the diſeaſe, the belly always became collapſed and hollow, with the ſkin wrinkled up into folds, and dry; the inteſtines felt through it like a maſs of ſoft clay, or inelaſtic ſubſtance; and their contents could be puſhed backwards and forwards through them, with a rumbling noiſe, indicating ſuch a relaxed and torpid ſtate of their coats, as no means could recover, if the habit had not been remarkably ſtrong and good before.

Several of the caſes ending in this way were opened at the hoſpital, and the general appearances were inflammation and thickening of ſome part of the inteftinal canal. Sometimes a degree of ulceration of the internal coat of the rectum, and adhefions of it to fome of the neighbouring parts, and moft commonly obftruction, and enlargement of the mefenteric glands, or enlarged and obftructed liver.

The rationale of this difeafe is perhaps as clear and fatisfactory as in any we meet with. It is a matter well eftablifhed from extenfive obfervation, that in all hot climates, and in India more than any, a fuperabundant and vitiated condition of the bilious fecretion, is in a manner a conftitutional temperament. In what manner this is produced, whether from a difeafed ftate of the organ itfelf, or from an alteration produced upon the fluid after its feparation in the liver, may not be fo eafy to determine. Perhaps both may have a fhare. A quantity of this difeafed bile getting into the ftomach very readily produces diforder there, and difturbs the functions of digeftion; and this, together with the accumulation of bile, and undigefted and difordered fluids, lodging in the turns of the duodenum, we confidered as fufficient to account for the fymptoms attending the firft first stage of the complaint; while irregular spasms, which generally affect the intestines, interrupt or prevent a free and regular passage downwards; and unless some purgative stimulus has been early and regularly employed, to carry off this load of bile, slime, and colluvies of diseased secretions, they soon run into a state of putrescent fermentation, which produces an acrimony sufficient to kindle up fever, and produce all the consequences we have mentioned. While this bilious redundancy continues, the functions of digestion, both in the stomach and upper tract of the intestines, are very imperfectly performed; and the long-continued irritation to which the intestines are subjected, comes at last to debilitate their tone and action, whereby they do not sufficiently propel their contents; and fresh accumulations and congestions are again and again formed, which, as they settle lower down, bring on a diseased state of the lower portion of the tract, particularly of the rectum, with topical affection of the gut. Though bilious plethora and fever, with the first set of affections have been all reduced; yet the long-continued irritation, together with debility and relaxation arising from the heat of the climate, has in a great meaſure deſtroyed the powers of digeſtion and chylifaction, ſo that no ſound and healthy nutriment is produced; or an obſtructed ſtate of the meſentery, or perhaps of the liver, has come on, which lays the foundation for maraſmus and a continual flux.

From this ſimple view of the diſeaſe, our plan of treatment was deduced, and conſiſted chiefly, or almoſt entirely, in the choice and exhibition of *evacuants*, adapted as well as we could to the condition of the diſorder, the ſtrength and conſtitution of the patient, and the irritability of the ſtomach and bowels, without a ſpecific regard to the fever, which we conſidered as ſymptomatic only. Notwithſtanding, however, of this ſimplicity of plan, it required all our caution and judgment to adapt theſe properly to the varying circumſtances and conditions of the patient, as well as in the proper choice of matters.

Cure.—The ſtate of the pulſe never ſeemed to indicate the neceſſity of letting blood. This was a remedy almoſt unknown with us; nor do I recollect ever to have wet a lancet in India, except in ſome caſes of acute hepatitis, or on account of ſome

ſome external injury. Inflammatory diatheſis, or a rigid and tenſe fibre, which Europeans may be ſuppoſed to retain for ſome time in hot climates, never appeared at all diſtinguiſhable in India. The long voyage, the greateſt part of it within the tropics, perhaps takes off that conſtitution by the time the India ſhores are reached.

When the fever was moderate, and the diſeaſe was not attended with much irritation of the ſtomach, pain, tenſion, or fulneſs of the abdomen, pretty briſk purgatives might be employed at firſt, and were neceſſary to unload the upper portions of the alimentary canal. But thoſe of the leaſt irritating ſort were always choſen, ſuch as Soluble Tartar *, with Manna; ſometimes with the addition of Tinct. Sennæ Comp., or, where more freedom could be uſed, Decoct. Tamarind. cum Senn.; or, in very irritable ſtates of the ſtomach, a ſaline mixture, with a large quantity of magneſia diffuſed in it, and three or four drachms of Tinct. Rhei, given by divided doſes. This made a very pleaſant and agreeable laxative, and always reſted on the ſtomach, eſpecially if made

* Tartris Potaſſæ.

warm with Ol. Menth. Pip., or with peppermint water. When the ſtomach had become ſettled and ſteady, and ſickneſs was abated, caſtor oil did as well as any. Emetics were never thought of, or the neutral ſalts, on account of their nauſeating effect. Weak chamomile tea, or rice-water only, were given to waſh the ſtomach when ſpontaneous vomiting took place. Perhaps, after bilious redundancy had been removed, and the diſeaſe had come to ſettle upon the colon and rectum, emetics, in mild and nauſeating doſes, or in full action, might have been uſeful, with a view to revulſion of ſecretions, and to promote the diſcharge by the ſkin, which, in theſe circumſtances, was always dry ; but this was not tried.

Plentiful dilution with farinaceous drinks, ſuch as rice-water, and frequent glyſtering, were very uſeful in relieving irregular ſpaſms and teneſmus, eſpecially on the days in which no purgative was uſed. Some purgative medicine, however, behoved to be given every ſecond or third day at leaſt, till the fever and griping, tumour and fulneſs of the abdomen went off, and the ſtools put on a healthy colour and appearance, or at leaſt nearly ſo ; for frequently a greeniſh caſt

of

of colour would remain in them, long after theſe ſymptoms were in a manner removed. In this condition, caſtor oil was frequently employed as a purge; and not only operated with as little ruffle and irritation as any, but brought off, perhaps, a fuller diſcharge from the upper part of the inteſtines than moſt. Decoction of Senna and Tamarinds, with a drachm or two of Sal Rochelle * diſſolved in it, was ſometimes employed. (The Soda Phoſphorata † was not then known at the hoſpital.) Some aromatic oil or ſeeds were generally added to whatever purge was made uſe of.

What I thought anſwered beſt, where a conſtant courſe of purging behoved to be kept up, either for the removal of bilious accumulations, or for counteracting irregular ſpaſms interrupting free paſſage, was about two drachms of cream of tartar ‡, with half an ounce of manna, boiled for ſome time in a conſiderable quantity of water, and ſome aromatic ſpirit added afterwards. This, taken in divided doſes, acted with leſs irritation,

I 4 and

* Tartris Potaſſæ et Sodæ.

† Phoſpas Sodæ.

‡ Supertartris Potaſſæ.

and weakened the patient lefs than moft we employed.

Under this treatment, the greateft number of our milder cafes recovered in the courfe of three weeks or a fortnight, without any further affiftance than perhaps fome light infufion of aromatics and bitters, after the bowel-diforder had fubfided.

When the attack was more fudden, with more fever and general commotion in the fyftem, with greater irritability of the ftomach, bowel-ficknefs, full, tenfe or tumid abdomen, fevere griping, heat, thirft and proftration of ftrength, we thought it neceffary to proceed with much greater caution.

For if, under fuch circumftances, any purge that acted brifkly was given, it was either rejected by the ftomach, or it brought on fo much retching and irritability, as was very difficultly allayed, or the fever, griping and pains of the abdomen were greatly exafperated by it. Often thofe of the mildeft kind could not be ventured on, till a quantity of the putrefcent fordes had been drawn off by the ufe of glyfters and plentiful dilution. But thefe, to be effectual, behoved to be given frequently in the fame day, and of confiderable quantity; ufing at firft plain rice-gruel, which we had always

always at hand, and afterwards adding a little Sal Glaub.*, as we ſaw needful. Rice-water was what we always gave for drink, with a little caſſia, ſometimes with tamarinds boiled in it; and often a quantity of magneſia was diffuſed in this, with directions to ſtir it when uſed.

If the patient was very hot and feveriſh, or had a vomiting, with ſome delirium, with much tenſion, fulneſs, and pain of the abdomen, or a weak and faultering pulſe, with coldneſs of the extremities, (in which ſtate we often found them), we thought it neceſſary to deſiſt, for ſome time, from giving any laxatives by the mouth, and truſted entirely to the uſe of glyſters: but then it was doubly neceſſary to be conſtant in the uſe of theſe, to ſupport the patient's ſtrength, and allay the irritability of the ſtomach, by ſuch cordials and anti-emetics as the little variety of a foreign hoſpital diſpenſatory put within our command; a little Madeira wine, boiled with caſſia, and given warm, or a little ſtrong tea, with Ol. Menth. Sativ.; or what anſwered as well as any thing, a mixture of Aq. Menth. Pip. or Sativ. with Tinct. Rhei and Magneſia,

* Sulphas Sodæ.

Magnefia, after every fit of retching; and in cafes of extreme irritability or weaknefs, 50 or 60 drops of laudanum, in a fmall glyfter. Given by the mouth, opium never appeared to be ufed either with fafety or advantage, or for any other purpofe, than merely as a palliative to gain time, or unlefs when joined with antimonial or ipecacuan wine in long ftanding diarrhœas.

The great danger to be apprehended in this difeafe, is from the readinefs with which inflammation and gangrene is brought on the inteftines, by irritation from acrid and putrid accumulations; and the only fecurity againft it lies in the timely and conftant ufe of proper evacuants, repeated as often as a return of fever, griping, pain and tenfion of the abdomen, foul tongue, bad tafte in the mouth, and impaired appetite, point out a renewal of thefe; and efpecially in guarding againft all irregularity and intemperance, whereby the original fymptoms are very readily recalled, fo that the fame ground has to be gone over and over again, in the fame complaint.

In fome inftances we had recoveries, where, from the feverity of fymptoms, continual vomitings, hiccup, cold fweats, weak pulfe, and the moft moſt putreſcent, offenſive and ſanious diſcharges by ſtool, there was every reaſon to conclude, that a degree of mortification had taken place in ſome portion of the inteſtines.

As an inſtance, I have put down the caſe of *John Quigly*, not in my own department of the hoſpital, but whom I ſaw frequently along with the gentleman who had charge of him; and who, by the conſtant and aſſiduous application of ſuch meaſures as have been mentioned, was perfectly recovered, and diſcharged cured. But the aggravating ſymptoms were two or three times renewed; and it behoved to keep up a conſtant purging by one means or other for the ſpace of a fortnight, before there was any amendment. Another inſtance, under my own care, was in the caſe of *John Bowerman*, who ſurvived, for a conſiderable length of time, the complete ſeparation of the whole rectum in a putrid bilious flux; and who, I made no doubt, might have fully recovered, had due care and attention been continued to him. His caſe is added.

Such was the general mode of treatment in what might be called the firſt ſtage of bilious fever and flux; and where there were no rooted obſtructions in the liver or meſentery, nor confirmed bilious diatheſis

diathesis previously existing, the disease most commonly terminated here. The fever, and that peculiar anxiety and oppression of spirits, which accompanies redundancy of bile in the upper part of the first passage, went gradually off. The stools returned to a natural colour and appearance; and the tongue and countenance put on a clear and healthy look.

But in a great proportion of cases the disease ran out to a great length beyond this, and commenced what might be called the *Second Stage*. The patient continued to be distressed with a continual flux, with straining, griping, mucous, and sometimes bloody stools; spasmodic pains in different parts of the abdomen; with heat and dry skin, and some evening fever. There was some return of appetite, or rather an anxious craving for something to fill up, and give a little tone and strength to the system; and though there was but little thirst, and the tongue looked pretty clean, yet there was no healthy digestion. There was some yellowness on the tongue towards the root, with a sallow and sickly cast of countenance, and dull yellowish colour in the white of the eye. Under these circumstances,

cumſtances, it was neceſſary to continue the uſe of purgatives at intervals, and to employ thoſe of a more active ſort. Whether it was, that few India fluxes of any ſtanding are not connected with ſome diſeaſe, or obſtructed ſtate of the liver or meſentery; or that ſome degree of this was induced in the courſe of bilious fluxes, I could not poſitively determine: but we conſtantly found, when the diſeaſe continued any time in this ſtate, mercurial purgatives anſwered much better than any other; or that mercury, combined with purgatives, and continued on the alterative plan; ſuch as a pill, compoſed of rhubarb, calomel, and ſoap, $1\frac{1}{2}$ gr. of each, given every night and morning, till it began to affect the mouth, effected cures when nothing elſe did any good; giving only now and then at night, when this did not keep the belly ſufficiently open, a pill with Aloes Socotorin. ſubſtituted in place of the rhubarb.

Whenever there was ſuſpicion of an inflammatory or obſtructed ſtate of the liver, the blue pills were given alone, till the mouth became affected, and theſe were continued for ſome time longer in milder doſes, interpoſing occaſional purgatives, when pain or griping gave reaſon to ſuſpect the renewal

renewal of fresh accumulations in any part of the canal. Under this mode of treatment, we were frequently succefsful, when we were gaining no ground, nor doing any good by evacuants and palliatives.

Mercurial friction we seldom had recourse to in these sort of cases; nor did we carry the use of mercury to such lengths as some pretend to have done for the cure of India fluxes, who seem to have proceeded without having had any determinate ideas about their nature, or the operation of mercury in their cure.

In the advanced, and especially in the last stage of this disease, tenesmus was apt to become a very troublesome symptom. Giving two or three pills a-day, composed of Pulv. Ipecac. gr. i., and Pulv. Rhei gr. iij. seldom failed to give relief; or what I sometimes substituted with the same effect was, Pulv. Ipecac., gr. iij.; Pulv. Crystal. Tart., gr. x.; Conserv. Rosarum, ʒij. made up into a bolus, and given in three equal parts through the day; and we made it a constant rule to add some aromatic oil, generally the Ol. Fœnicul. Dulc. to all our alterative and purgative pills.

Whenever

Whenever ſevere pain and gri ing, with ſoreneſs to the touch, or tenſion in a y particu'ar part of the abdomen, took place, and continued fixed to a ſpot, and was not fully removed by free and full evacuation, eſpecially if along with theſe ſymptoms, the parietes of the abdomen were tenſe and retracted towards the back-bone; great and immediate relief was obtained by the application of a large bliſter over the affected part. This we had ſometimes occaſion to repeat again and again in the courſe of the ſame complaint, and often thought the patient was relieved by it from the moſt imminent danger; in ſo much that it became a kind of routine of practice with us in ſuch like caſes, if there was a fixed pain in any particular part of the abdomen, and repeated evacuations and fomenting the belly did not ſucceed in removing it, eſpecially if this was accompanied with heat, tenſion and retraction of the teguments, or whenever, in the progreſs of the diſorder, a new affection of this kind came on,—immediately to apply a large bliſter over the part; and when ſevere griping pains came to affect the lower belly and top of the rectum, with ſtraining and bloody ſtools, ftools, we applied them above the pubes with the fame advantage.

With regard to the dietetic part of practice, an hofpital admitted of but little choice or variety; nor could ftrict attention be had to this on fuch an eftablifhment, except upon a general plan. But with regard to officers, and fuch as were at fick quarters, we made it a general rule to forbid all hot broths, tea or foups, and roafted meat. What feemed to agree beft with every body where animal food could be made ufe of, was the native mode of dreffing it: The *pillaws* and *curries*, or grilled fowls, with native pepper, and chicken-broth with the fame feafoning. Fat and roafted meats were ftrictly forbidden. Dried white fifh and water for breakfaft anfwered very well, and a glafs or two of Madeira, or brandy and water after dinner. In the fecondary ftages, we never forbade the ufe of fruits, efpecially fuch as were aftringent; as the mango, and guavo or pomegranate; and we always directed a part of the rind to be eaten along with them. They were grateful and ufeful antifeptics; only, much of the pomegranate

rind

rind was too ſtrongly aſtringent to be uſed indiſcriminately *.

In the ſecondary ſtages of this diſeaſe, we found, that the exhibition of opium, in the form of glyſter, could be admitted of, and was frequently of ſervice in relieving pain and teneſmus, and in procuring quiet and eaſy nights, and thereby recruiting the ſtrength; but it never did good in any other way, or while bilious accumulations prevailed; and it behoved to be alternated with purgatives.

In but too many caſes where the conſtitution had been much enfeebled and relaxed, or the ſtrength exhauſted by previous diſeaſe; inſtead of procuring a termination of the flux, we ſaw it become more frequent. The bilious colour diſappeared from the ſtools, and they became white and

 mucous.

* The author of theſe obſervations was reduced to as low a ſtate by bilious flux as ever any European in India. The firſt turn towards recovery was found at the hoſpitable tables of Vizagapatam, where all the tropical fruits were in plenty. Nature and appetite prompted ſtrongly, and the fulleſt indulgence was followed, not only with impunity, but with manifeſt advantage.

mucous. The tongue got clean, but a fallow look remained. There was no return of healthy appetite, but a degree of hectic fever continued, with progreffive lofs of flefh and ftrength ; and the food paffed through the bowels in an indigefted ftate ; the difeafe terminating in its *Third and Laft Stage,*—a continual flux or lienteric diarrhœa. In this condition, neither bark, opium, nor tonics, were of any fervice. Bark, in fome inftances, rather feemed to do harm. Now and then, cures were effected by a flow and gradual courfe of the blue pill, affifted with rhubarb and bitters, with aromatic feeds infufed in brandy and water. Perhaps in fuch cafes, naufeating dofes of antimonials, or occafional full vomiting might have been of ufe; and mercurial frictions might have been preferable to the pills, but we had fo much experience of the good effects of thefe, without aggravating the bowel diforder, that inunction was but feldom tried.

Fifteen or fixteen drops of Elix. Vitriol. in a large draught of weak infufion of the *Margofa* leaf, was always grateful to the ftomach, and improved the appetite. Neither the Quaffia Simarouba nor Cafcarilla barks were in the hofpital, nor did

did they ſeem to be much known in India practice. In the advanced ſtages of bilious fluxes where the ſyſtem was much reduced and relaxed by the diſeaſe, many officers found benefit from the uſe of a *long* ſhawl wrapped round the abdomen next the ſkin; and others who could not afford the expence, found the ſame advantage from a flannel bandage.

Both in the bilious and liver fluxes, where we had occaſion to adminiſter long and repeated courſes of mercury, I obſerved, that it was longer, in whatever way employed, of affecting the mouth, and that ptyaliſm ſeldom could be carried the ſame length by it as in colder countries; and ſo far from weakening the habit, inducing hectic, and a diſſolved ſtate of the blood, our patients generally got full and plump after its uſe; inſomuch, that we ſometimes looked on this as the ſureſt indication of its having been effectual for removing the diſeaſe for which it was employed.

We have already mentioned the general appearances found on diſſecting ſuch as died of bilious fever and flux. To have been more particular would have thrown little additional light on the ſubject. The following caſe, though not ſtrictly connected with the disease we have treated of, it may be worth while to put down, as tending to show the dangerous tendency of bowel-diseases in India; and how readily inflammation and gangrene are brought on the intestines from causes which are seldom, in Europe, productive of such effects.

DISSECTION.

On the 4th of August 1782, was admitted into the hospital, *A. B.* seaman, under thirty years of age, affected with fever, small, weak and frequent pulse, and pain of the abdomen; but without tension or fulness. He was under some delirium, and his countenance was pale, with cold sweats over his limbs. His respiration was laboured and irregular; with much anxiety in his countenance, and jactation of his body and limbs. He said what he ate and drank did not pass through him, and he complained of much pain on pressing the umbilical region. Warm fomentations were applied to the abdomen, and some glysters were prescribed for him in the evening, and through the night; but nothing was brought away but slimy mucus, with much straining. Next morning a laxative

laxative was given him, but was not retained on his ftomach. There was more delirium, or rather wildnefs of look and gefture, for at times he fpoke very collectedly. Pulfe very weak and quick, with cold fweats, conftant jactation and reftlefsnefs. All his drink was fpouted up as foon as it reached his ftomach, but without retching or hiccup. After renewing the fomenting, and a glyfter, two pills, containing ten grains of calomel and a grain of opium were given him, and retained on his ftomach; but without producing any effect, and he died in the courfe of the following night.

On opening his body next afternoon, the omentum was found very much thickened; the lower border of it inflamed and red. The whole of it was dragged over to the left fide, where it was crammed in between the inteftines and parietes of the abdomen. The whole track of the ilium was inflamed, and its blood-veffels enlarged and full of blood. Where it enters the colon, were found coiled up two large lumbrici worms, alive when taken out. Over thefe, the coats of the inteftine were thickened and inflamed to a high degree, and much contracted in diameter, but with no erofion or ulceration of the gut.

In the ilium above, were two diſtinct intus-ſuſceptions, each of four inches in length, the ſuperior portions inverted within the inferior. The included parts were pale and bloodleſs. The colon was empty and flaccid. There were no appearances of bilious accumulations, or other marks of diſeaſe.

CASE OF MORTIFIED RECTUM.

James Bowerman, invalid, ſome time in the beginning of November 1782, complained of a looſeneſs, with gripes and teneſmus, which he ſaid had come on ſome days before, but which he had not mentioned ſooner, in expectation of its ſoon going off. He had been in good health, and the wound for which he had been invalided had been long healed up. On inſpecting his ſtools, they were of a dark colour, and very offenſive to the ſmell. His pulſe was frequent, with heat of his ſkin, pain and tenſion of the abdomen, and ſome difficulty of voiding his urine. His tongue foul, and countenance ſallow.

His

His abdomen was well fomented, and a dofe of foluble tartar and manna was immediately given him, affifted by frequent glyfters, whereby much dark-coloured fetid ftuff was brought away. This courfe was continued for four days fucceffively, without the colour or fetor of the difcharge being in the leaft altered. But the difficulty of voiding urine had increafed; and for the laft twenty-four hours he had paffed only a fmall quantity, equal to a few fpoonfuls, with great ftraining and pain. There was fome fulnefs above the os pubis, but not like that occafioned by the retention of much urine in the bladder. A catheter was, however, paffed, and went eafily, but no urine was found in it. A glyfter, with forty drops of Spirit. Terebinth. was given him in the evening; and two tea-fpoonfuls of Spirit. Nitri Dulc. were put into his drink through the night. He paffed at different times, before ten o'clock next day, about a pint of urine, but with much pain and ftraining. Still there was a good deal of fever, with general fwelling and uneafinefs of the abdomen. Only cordial foup, and fome wine, were given him for this day.

On the eighth and tenth day from his complaint, the physic was repeated, with a plain glyster at night, and the abdomen was fomented once every day. After this, he continued to pass his urine freely.

On the eleventh, there was no amendment; his pulse was still quick and feeble; and the appearance of his stools nothing better. This day he complained of a pain about the anus, which had prevented him from receiving the glyster last night. On inspection, the edge of the gut was found to be swelled out all round, and much inflamed. The verge of the passage was of a deep red colour, with a thin ichorous matter draining from it. Bark and wine were now given him in large doses, and a poultice was applied over the swelling. By next morning, the whole was black and mortified. At night, the whole of the rectum was found hanging inverted from the anus nearly seven inches in length; the greatest part in a mortified state, but here and there the different coats distinguishable, and easily separated from each other. This was all removed; and after washing and fomenting the parts with chamomile decoction, the poultice was continued over the

the opening. The following day, ſome detached portions of the gut came away. Still there was conſiderable pain and tenſion of the abdomen, with a low and weak pulſe; but he kept up his ſpirits remarkably well. The inteſtinal diſcharge came away inſenſibly, with a great deal of ſanious and putrid ſloughs from the ſides of the opening, which made a frequent renewal of the poultices neceſſary; and every time this was done, a large ſyringe-full of warm water, with a little Port wine, or Mel Roſarum, was thrown up. To the fourth day from the ſeparation of the gut, there was but little change, only the diſcharge was not ſo much diſcoloured, and his belly was conſiderably eaſier. The external edge of the opening was ſtill black, and much ſwelled out; but within there was an appearance of its caſting off. In three days more, this was effected; leaving a monſtrous opening, large enough to introduce a gooſe's egg with eaſe. But all within, to the top of the ſacrum, or as far as the eye could reach, the ſides of the opening were perfectly clean, with a kindly ſuppuration and granulations ſpringing up. The appearance of the alvine diſcharge was by this time much mended, and nearly of a natural colour. The ſtate

of

of the abdomen became much eaſier; his pulſe fuller, and his looks better. The poultices and ſyringing the ſore were now laid aſide, and only a little dry lint was laid lightly into the opening, with a large ſpread pledget over it, to exclude the air; and this was renewed four times in the twenty-four hours. His bark and wine were ſtill continued; but it was neceſſary to interpoſe a laxative every third day, otherwiſe his belly became tenſe and painful.

In this way he went on for fourteen days from the ſeparation of the gut, with every appearance in his favour. The fever and flux, pain and uneaſineſs in the abdomen, had been entirely removed. Urine always paſſed freely, and without pain, and he had recovered his appetite and a conſiderable degree of ſtrength, when I was diſabled by ſickneſs from attending the hoſpital. Soon after this he had become worſe, and was complaining again of pain and tenſion in the abdomen; and I underſtood that his phyſic had not been regularly continued, but in place of it opiates to allay pain and procure ſleep. On the 4th of December, on ſending again to inquire for him, I was informed, the pain of his bowels had entirely left

left him, though his belly was much ſwelled, and that he had but little diſcharge by ſtool; that his looks were bad, and his pulſe very low and weak. From this account, it was eaſy to foretell his fate, which the ſame night concluded, happily, perhaps, for himſelf; though I once conſidered him as a gained caſe, and was anxiouſly contriving the beſt means for preſerving the paſſage, and how the diſtreſs of a conſtant *ſtillicidium alvinum* might be beſt prevented.

SOME OBSERVATIONS ON THE OTHER BILIOUS DISEASES OF INDIA.

TRUE and formed jaundice occurred at the hoſpital, in ſome inſtances, where the whole ſkin, eyes and urine, were tinged with a deep yellow colour. This appeared, in all the caſes, to ariſe from a redundancy of bile, without being attended with obſtruction of the gall-ducts.

It was ſoon and eaſily removed in them all by a few purges, compoſed of mercury, ſquills and ſoap,

ſoap, followed by the exhibition of bitters. But where any degree of fever or quickneſs of pulſe were preſent, two or three doſes of Soluble Tartar, and Manna with Tinct. Rhei, were always premiſed.

Ten or twelve caſes of intermittent fever were met with; but there was not one of them that did not ariſe from diſorder or redundancy of the bilious ſecretion, or from obſtructed viſcera. The type was regular in none. Quotidians changed into tertians, and *vice verſâ.* The intermiſſions were not perfect. The patient complained of headach, want of appetite, oppreſſion of ſpirits, nauſea and griping pains, or had an irregular flux; ſometimes a hard or tender liver.

No perfect or laſting cures were made by bark, unleſs a long courſe of purging had gone before it. It had more or leſs effect in ſtopping, or ſuſpending the fits for a time; but very often it only rendered them more irregular, or, what was worſe, it changed the diſeaſe into a continued fever.

It was not thought ſafe or proper in any caſe, to exhibit bark without a frequent alternation of purgatives, or without being combined with aromatic

matic ſeeds, and vitriolated or ſoluble tartar. In one caſe of regular tertian, which was ſuppoſed to be ſimple, it was thought the bark had made a perfect cure, and the patient was diſcharged under that idea: but he was returned to us not many days after, under a moſt violent bilious fever; with tumor, tenſion, fulneſs and heat of the abdomen, loaded yellow tongue, and ſuch a degree of wild delirium, as rendered him perfectly unmanageable, ſo that little or nothing could be done for him; and he died in two days after his ſecond admiſſion, —a ſure proof that the ſource of his diſeaſe was deeper than had been at firſt ſuſpected.

In moſt inſtances, this diſeaſe was removed by a courſe of purging alone: or, if it proved obſtinate, eſpecially if the liver or belly felt hard, or enlarged or tender to the touch, a courſe of mercurial alteratives, with purges occaſionally interpoſed, was certainly ſucceſsful.

DISEASES OF THE THORACIC VISCERA.

Such caſes were exceedingly rare, or rather never appeared at all under an idiopathic form. Pulmonary conſumption was wholly unknown.

There

There were ſeveral caſes, where matter collected in the liver, eroded the diaphragm, and the lungs were waſted, and ſpit up by coughing. Only two caſes of catarrh, with cough, and ſymptoms threatening pneumonia, by being neglected, were met with ; but both of them were eaſily cured by bliſtering, and the common remedies for that affection.

RETURN FROM INDIA IN THE MEDEA FRIGATE.

FOR a conſiderable period after leaving the Indian ſeas, a tendency to the diſeaſes of that climate, and a bilious diatheſis, were obſervable among the ſeamen.

We had ſimple bilious fluxes ; fluxes connected with old ſtanding obſtructions of the liver and meſentery ; and a few caſes of acute hepatitis.

The captain's ſteward had long laboured under one of theſe old ſtanding obſtructions of the liver, which do not readily terminate in acute inflammation, but which are often attended with long-continued

tinued ill health; and produce occaſionally very untractable and dangerous diſorders. He had been on ſhore attending on his worthy and benevolent maſter, Captain, (now Admiral) Sir Eraſmus Gower, where, to his other misfortunes, he had contrived to add a confirmed pox. When he came on board, he was attacked with bilious vomitings, and an irregular flux, and was altogether in ſo reduced and impaired a ſtate, that little was expected to be done for him, beyond palliating his complaints. As we approached the Cape, his diſeaſe put on the form of a tertian intermittent; with the fits at firſt pretty regular; but they became leſs ſo as the diſeaſe advanced. They were ſo violent as to make it doubtful, whether he might ſupport them long, unleſs they could be mitigated. A mild emetic, and ſeveral purges of ſoluble tartar with manna and magneſia, were preſcribed for him; and at laſt recourſe was had to bark, with vitriolated tartar, and infuſion of chamomile. This ſuſpended the fits for a week; but at the end of that time he did not look better, and they returned with greater violence than ever. After a few repetitions, the diſeaſe changed into a continued fever, with a putrid bilious flux, which laſted for two months.

His

His ſtools were at firſt thin; almoſt black, highly offenſive to the ſmell, and attended with much pain, tumor and hardneſs of the belly. But he never complained of any pain in the region of the liver, unleſs when it was hard preſſed; though it was certain the foundation of the whole lay there. By the time the ſhip reached England, which was in exactly four months from our leaving Madras, his complaints had been in a great meaſure removed. His ſtools had become nearly natural; his countenance was putting on by degrees the look of health, which it had long wanted; and he had recovered his appetite and ſo much ſtrength as to be able to walk the decks.

The treatment of this caſe was throughout the ſame as we followed in the India bilious fluxes; with only this difference in the choice of laxatives, that a ſaline mixture, with about half a grain of tartar emetic, in divided doſes through the day, was frequently employed, and anſwered the purpoſe of moving his bowels as well as any. Great and repeated benefit was alſo derived from bliſtering the abdomen, whenever ſevere pain and griping, referred to a particular ſpot, gave reaſon to ſuſpect the exiſtence of topical affection there.

The

The only radical cure for his complaints would have been a gentle and long-continued courſe of mercury; and this could now have been undertaken with ſafety: but the ſhip being to be paid off, he was ſent to Haſlar Hoſpital, where he did not long ſurvive.

GENERAL OBSERVATIONS.

In many late communications from India, we find Dysentery (of which we have ſaid nothing) ſo frequently ſpoken of as one of the common and ordinary diſeaſes of the country, and without any thing ſtated to diſtinguiſh it from this diſeaſe, as it appears elſewhere, and has been deſcribed by former writers, as to render it neceſſary to ſubjoin ſome obſervations to explain how this has happened; and alſo to ſhew, why here, and no where elſe, mercury and the nitric acid have been employed, and with ſo much ſucceſs, in its cure.

By conſulting Dr Clark's Remarks on the Diſeaſes of India, and two Memoirs on the Health of the 88th Regiment, by Dr Macgregor, publiſhed

 in

in Dr Duncan's Annals, and in the third Number of the Phyfical and Surgical Journal, we find from their diffections in the complaint which they uniformly call *Dyfentery*, the very fame difeafed appearances as were difcovered by us on diffecting the bodies of thofe who died of bilious and liver diforders; viz. inflamed or ulcerated liver, a difeafed ftate of the mefenteric glands; inflammation and thickening of the inteftines, with effufions of blood between their coats; erofion, ulceration of the internal membrane, and fometimes fphacelus and gangrene. But with dyfentery, as it appears in all other countries, liver-difeafe is rarely found connected; and the inteftinal affection is in a much inferior degree, or confined more to the internal membrane.

They defcribe the ftools as being copious and liquid; frequently bilious; and never as containing fcybalæ. Dr Macgregor fays, " In 500 ca-" fes, he does not think that fcybalæ were paffed " in fix of them." This difeafed condition of the inteftines, and the dyfenteric fymptoms which fometimes took place to a confiderable degree in all bilious fluxes, we confidered as the natural and neceffary confequences of difeafed bile and vitiated

ted ſecretions, acting on parts highly irritable, and therefore much diſpoſed to diſeaſe, as almoſt the whole abdominal viſcera ſeem to be in India. Topical diſeaſe of the liver, we did not conſider as a cauſe of fluxes, or of dyſenteric ſypmptoms in them, in any other way than as giving occaſion to vitiated and depraved ſecretions. But a ſufficient diſtinction is in my opinion to be made between the *bilious* and *hepatic fluxes* of India, and *dyſentery*, from the following conſiderations.

In thoſe that depend on ſimple diſorder of the ſecretions, and where the liver is not primarily affected, there is always much more diſturbance and diſorder in the functions of the ſtomach, and upper part of the inteſtinal canal,—bilious vomitings and dejections, with ſtomach and bowel ſickneſs,—than takes place in dyſentery; and the diſeaſe reſembles much more cholera morbus.

The diſeaſe ſometimes terminates, and health is reſtored, by the firſt evacuations, without dyſenteric ſymptoms ever appearing, or it runs on to ſpeedy inflammation and gangrene, with a putrid bilious flux; and although in ſuch fluxes, there is generally ſome fever preſent, it is only acceſſary or accidental, and is never of any regular type or du-

 ration.

ration. The ſtools are generally of a deep yellow or green colour, and ſeldom, in the early part of the diſorder, mucous; nor is teneſmus ever an early ſymptom. For the moſt part, they are eaſily procured by the gentleſt laxatives; and when not interrupted by abdominal ſpaſms, copious and liquid, never ſcybalous: and that kind of dyſentery which ariſes in camps, hoſpitals, and crowded ſhips, is diſtinguiſhed from all other fluxes, in being highly infectious; whereas thoſe of India, by all concurring accounts, are never ſo in any degree. Fluxes properly hepatic have the ſymptoms ſomewhat varied, but are clearly referable to a diſtinct affection different from the dyſenteric.

Whether dyſentery, under its true and proper form, be a native diſeaſe of India, or of any tropical country; or if it ever appears in them without being imported from colder latitudes, I am not prepared to ſay. In crowded ſhips, or in ſimilar ſituations, it may perhaps be generated, (eſpecially among people newly from Europe) any where. But I am not diſpoſed to think it a coaſt diſeaſe of India. That which aroſe in the fleet that ſailed from England under the command of Commodore Johnſtone,

gave

gave place to other diseases long before we reached the Indian seas.

In Dr Macgregor's first report, it is stated, "That the diseases far most prevalent" (on the Bombay coast) "and the most deserving of serious notice, have been dysentery and hepatitis; "and if not the same disease, the two are most "clearly allied in this country. Five hundred "and forty-four cases occurred during the year "1801, and of these, forty died. The bodies of "twenty-two were inspected after death, and the "liver was found diseased in sixteen." It is from this inspection that we are informed, that "dysentery is almost always connected with a disease of "the liver as a cause." Yet it is afterwards said, that "in other cases, the liver was found but "slightly, or not at all affected;" but the morbid intestinal affections we have mentioned, were found in all of them. With regard to the cure, speaking of both under one head, viz. hepatitis and dysentery, it is said, "A large proportion of the cases "were cured by remedies that have never been "supposed to operate on the liver. But it must be "confessed," (he adds) "that our cures by these "remedies were more frequent and certain, soon

" after our arrival in India, than they of late have " been." The remedies employed for the firſt three months are enumerated, and it is ſtated, that they were uſed with conſiderable ſucceſs; but it immediately follows, " Yet we ſoon found, that " mercury and analagous remedies," (viz. the nitric acid) " were to be the moſt generally relied " on."

Much more to the ſame purpoſe, will be found in Dr Macgregor's Second Memoir, and in Dr Clark's Remarks; ſufficient we think to warrant the concluſion, that the diſeaſe which they uniformly called Dyſentery in India, is in its nature, ſymptoms, proximate cauſe, and alſo in its method of cure, entirely different from that which has been deſcribed under this name in all other countries; that it differs in nothing from bilious and liver-fluxes, ſo commonly to be met with there; and that if this name is to be applied, it ought to be joined with one which may ſerve to diſtinguiſh the diſeaſe from other varieties,—ſuch as the *Hepatic* or *Bilious Dyſentery of India.*

From the known effects of mercury in the cure of liver-diſeaſes, and in the removal of meſenteric obſtructions, we will have an eaſy explanation, why,

why, in all ſevere caſes of dyſentery as it appears in India, mercury and the nitric acid were to be the moſt generally relied on for their removal.

How far theſe remedies, in moderate doſes, may be found innocent, or uſeful for the cure of real dyſentery, or in all its combinations, I do not undertake to ſay; but I am perſuaded, if given in doſes that have been preſcribed for what has gone under that name in India, they could not fail in many inſtances to be exceedingly hurtful.

In fluxes purely bilious, I ſometimes thought that mercury even produced good effects as a ſimple corrector, from an alteration for the better being not unfrequently made by it on the alvine diſcharges, before it could have entered the ſyſtem in ſuch quantity, as to affect the ſtate of the organs concerned.

Both Drs Macgregor, Clark and Chryſtie agree in ſtating, that dyſentery is never contagious in India. I obſerved no evidence of the exiſtence of this in any of the diſeaſes to be met with there; and I am doubtful, whether, with the exception of the exanthemata which appear to be ſo in every country, there be any others of that deſcription.

This, were it confirmed, might appear a ſtriking peculiarity, ſince we know that in countries under a ſimilar latitude, and under a ſimilar degree of heat, ſome of the moſt active and virulent contagions, are in a manner endemic; and are ſuppoſed only to appear in colder climates by tranſportation. Thus, Yellow Fever has become endemic in the Weſt Indies, and the Plague in Egypt and the Levant. But plagues and contagions appear to have been in former times equally common to all the countries of Europe; and there are ſome reaſons to conclude, that the yellow fever was firſt imported to the Weſt India iſlands from the ſouthern States of America. The Turks are but a late colony from the north of Aſia, and the population of the Weſt Indies is conſtantly recruited by ſupplies from Europe or North America. It is well aſcertained, that theſe contagious diſeaſes produce the ſevereſt effects upon new comers, or perſons whoſe ſyſtem of fibres has not been ſubdued and relaxed by a reſidence in a hot climate, but from the nature of the countries in which theſe diſeaſes have become fixed, and from the ſeaſon of the year, viz. the autumnal, at which the contagion ſpreads and becomes moſt active, there

is

is ſome reaſon for ſuppoſing that both plague, yellow fever, and perhaps the late Cadiz, Malaga and Gibraltar fevers, though each poſſeſſing a ſpecific contagion *ſui generis*, may yet have ſo far a common character, that it is contagion combined with, or engrafted on a bilious diatheſis, or vitiated ſtate of this ſecretion: Hence, perhaps, the reaſon why ſome of them are to be found at all ſeaſons of the year, in countries where this is a conſtitutional temperament; and the difference, and even oppoſition in the plans of cure that have been followed, has neceſſarily ariſen from the variety that takes place in relation to climate, ſeaſon, and the ſtate of the weather, as diſpoſing more or leſs to bilious redundancy, inflammatory diatheſis, a rich and denſe blood, or a rigid ſyſtem of fibres.

One reaſon why contagious diſeaſes prevail leſs in India than in other ſimilar latitudes, may perhaps be the greater diſtance from Europe; the long tract of navigation moſtly within the tropics, which allows time for diſſipating all ſeeds of contagion from that quarter, and for taking off the temperament of body moſt congenial to it, and for aſſimilating the habit to what is the morbid conſtitution of the country. Should ſuch diſeaſes ever become

become endemic there, the probability is, they will be imported from the north.

It remains to ſubjoin ſome obſervations on Bilious and Liver Diſeaſes, as they appear in our own country.

To a ſtranger, the diſtinguiſhing ſymptoms of liver inflammation in India appear at firſt not a little obſcure, from the prominency of the ſecondary and ſymptomatic affections with which it is generally attended. In Europe, the difficulty is rather increaſed from their variety. Here we often meet with pulmonary affection combined with it, to ſuch a degree as to render it difficult for us to ſay which is the radical and which the ſympathetic diſorder; and wherever there is much delicacy of conſtitution or phthiſical tendency in the habit, we are always uncertain of which the danger may be the greater; or how far the meaſures we employ for the removal of diſeaſe in the one organ, may not foſter or aggravate that in the other. The diſeaſe is in general more of a chronic nature. A variety of ſymptoms, referable to other heads, as thoſe of dyſpepſia, hypochondriaſis, and what are called the nervous affections, are ſure to combine with

with it ; and the radical diſeaſe is often ſo ſlightly marked, as to render it not a little difficult to ſay what or which is the principal or primary among them.

Bilious redundance and depravations, which give a ſtanding character to many of the India diſeaſes, are there alſo pretty diſtinctly pointed out, from the appearance of the excretions, and from the colour of the tongue, eyes and urine.

Many European diſorders have the ſame origin ; but the marks of it are not ſo well expreſſed, or they are of a more temporary ſtanding ; or the ſame cauſe is found to operate in a different manner, and to produce more varieties.

Of theſe, it may be ſufficient to notice the following.

Perſons returning from either India, often bring home with them a conſtitution, waſted and debilitated by the diſeaſes of thoſe climates ; from which they recover with difficulty, or not at all. It is not, however, often that a ſimple bilious diatheſis continues long at home, where there are no obſtructions in the liver or meſentery ; and perſons who have been waſted and reduced to the laſt degree by India fluxes, ſometimes recover perfectly at at home, and enjoy good health, and as firm a ſtate of the ſtomach and bowels as ever.

A diſpoſition to redundancy of the bilious ſecretion, and to cholera morbus, is obſervable during the autumnal months, in all the ſouthern countries of Europe. The diſeaſe is, in general, very manageable, under the uſe of the ſame remedies as we employed in the milder bilious fluxes of India. Small doſes of ipecacuanha and rhubarb are very uſeful; and the beſt form of theſe is when made into ſmall pills. Doſes of ſoda phoſphorata, given in beef-tea, form one of the mildeſt and moſt lenient laxatives we can employ, unleſs in very irritable ſtates of the ſtomach. It is not very certain in its operation as a purgative; but in repeated ſmall doſes, is the beſt laxative we can uſe in all caſes where blood is paſſed with the ſtools. Rhubarb and Pulvis antimonialis mixed together, may be employed for the ſame purpoſe; or, what anſwers as certainly as any, when the ſtomach is unſettled, a ſaline mixture with calcined magneſia diffuſed in it. A proportion of tincture of jalap added to this mixture and well ſweetened, makes a very effectual purge, and is one as eaſily exhibited to children as any I have tried. Plentiful

tiful dilution is a material part of the treatment. Opiates are but little wanted, and the premature uſe of them is often hurtful.

In ſome habits, we find a conſtitutional tendency to bilious diſeaſe, operating entirely in a different way, and which is often of long ſtanding. It is moſt common to females about the middle or advance of life, but never remains to old age. Far from inducing purging, the bile takes a contrary direction, and, by regurgitating into the ſtomach, occaſions headachs, ſickneſs, depreſſion of ſpirits, with nauſea and bilious vomitings. This comes at irregular, ſometimes at lengthened intervals; laſts for one, two or three days, and then goes off, ſometimes with, but often without, a bilious purging, and without much injury to the health, till the return of another fit.

I have never ſucceeded in doing any thing material to correct this diſpoſition. Keeping an open belly is always of conſequence; as the patients are diſpoſed to be coſtive, even while under the complaint. For this, I have found a pill compoſed of equal parts of aloes, jalap, and calomel, or of Extract. Colocynth. comp. *Ph. Lond.* with calomel, two or three for a doſe, anſwer well. And

ſome

ſome patients have found benefit from uſing equal parts of Pulv. Rhei, Magneſia uſta, Flor. Chamæmel. and Rad. Zinziber., as much every day, or every other day, as opens the belly gently.

Such diſorders as have been mentioned, may all be referred to ſimple redundancy or regurgitation of bile, but little vitiated or altered in its quality. But there are others to be met with, which ſeem to originate in highly depraved ſtates of this fluid, together with indigeſta or diſordered aliments operating lower down in the alimentary canal, but attended alſo with much ſtomach diſorder, and which are ſometimes carried to a very dangerous and fatal height. This, too, occurs moſt frequently to females, eſpecially to thoſe who are ſubject to coſtiveneſs, and to diſorder in the digeſtive organs; to what they call *ſtomach cholics;* to acid eructations, and dyſpepſia. They are ſeized with a ſevere pain referred to the region of the ſtomach, the left ſide, or upper part of the abdomen, often without any warning, and with ſpaſmodic ſtricture, or what they call a *ſevere cramp pain.* On examination, the muſcles of the abdomen are ſometimes found to be ſpaſmodically affected, and it is ſtrongly retracted. Severe retching and vomitings come

come on. The ejecta, ſometimes bilious, but oftener highly acid, or of a pungent and acrimonious taſte and ſmell. In the worſt ſort of caſes, there is great ſickneſs, with debility, and a weak faultering pulſe ; faintings and coldneſs of the extremities, with a pale hippocratic countenance from the very firſt. The ſpaſmodic affection, perhaps, goes off, and the abdomen rather becomes tumid and painful, with flatulent diſtention and borborygmi. Sometimes the patient is cut off in this way before the bowels are fully moved, to aſcertain the ſtate of their contents. In caſes leſs ſevere, and where this is effected, the evacuations are offenſive to the ſmell, green, fetid or ſanious, and the complaint is removed by a courſe of purging. Where death takes place ſuddenly, the perſon is generally ſuppoſed to have been cut off by gout, or by cramp in the ſtomach. Enteritis or ilius do not attack ſo very rapidly, nor do they prove ſo ſpeedily fatal ; and it is not conceived, that bile or indigeſta, confined in any part of the alimentary canal, can acquire an acrimony that ſhall produce ſuch effects at once, and without much previous warning.

But

But this is not the only caſe in which we find that the cauſes of diſeaſe do not produce their effects till they are accumulated to a certain force. Nature will do much to reſiſt or obviate impreſſions that are hurtful, provided ſhe is not ſurpriſed and overwhelmed at once. How ſhe effects this reſiſtance in the caſe before us, admits of an eaſier explanation than we are able to give in many others. The firſt paſſages are all lined with a ſlimy mucus, to defend them from acrimony. An increaſe of this ſecretion will take place, wherever, in any of the turns of the inteſtine, acrimonious indigeſta begin to be accumulated. When theſe come to be carried ſuddenly forward to another portion of the canal, it is then only the full effect will be produced. We had occaſion to ſee this often verified in the bilious diſeaſes of India, where we were ſometimes well aſſured of the exiſtence of highly acrimonious accumulations in the turns of the inteſtines. The patient would have but little or no pain, griping, or ſickneſs, while his bowels were kept quiet and undiſturbed by purgatives; but the moment their contents were put in motion, every thing was ſuddenly reverſed, and the patient was ſometimes as quickly and effectually killed by it, it, as if a ſtrong ſedative poiſon had been artificially injected into his inteſtines. Every perſon, ſome time in his life, may have felt what will ſerve to confirm what we are endeavouring to illuſtrate. Something has been eaten which has diſagreed with the ſtomach; that is to ſay, has not taken on the proper chylifactive digeſtion, but has undergone ſome other change, and generated an acrimonious mixture; and ſome of the ſevereſt caſes of the diſorder we are deſcribing, can be plainly referred to this cauſe. Nothing perhaps is felt till the next day, or later. Sharp cholic pains, accompanied with bowel-ſickneſs, and with a ſenſe of motion through the guts, begin to be felt. This proceeds lower and lower down, till a few looſe ſtools removes the whole. The origin of the complaint is made evident, in other caſes, from griping pain, and a feculent purging, having preceded the attack. This will be ſuſpended during the ſeverity of the ſtomach affection and the ſpaſms, but is renewed again when theſe go off; and the complaint is removed by the aſſiſtance of purgatives. We are in danger of being miſled by the ſpaſms, which the patient himſelf refers to the ſtomach and internal parts; but in this he is miſtaken. They affect only the abdominal mufcles, and are only fymptomatic, arifing from irritation in a diftant part; juft as happens in tetanus, or as we found them in the *mort de chien*. The offending matters are not in this cafe lodged there, but in the turns of the duodenum or jejunum, and the ftomach acts readily in ejecting the contents, and admits of being filled with drinks, which it could not be, were it fpafmodically contracted. Filling the ftomach with warm weak tea, is often of fervice in abating the pain and fpafms.

Another way in which we are ready to deceive ourfelves, if we are not on our guard, is by diffections. The patient dies. The body is permitted to be opened, and this it is fuppofed is to explain every thing. This is done 48 hours perhaps, or longer after death. The turns of the inteftines, or fome portions of them, appear fuffufed and red, or approaching to a purple colour, with the coats thickened, and the mefenteric veffels turgid; all this heightened by the contraction of parts, and coagulation of the blood, which takes place after death. Thefe are fuppofed to be the effects of inflammation, and the patient is thought to have died of enteritis. But the cafe is totally different. Inflammation

mation of the inteſtines is quite a different thing, and never proves ſo quickly fatal. Theſe appearances are all the effects, and not the cauſe of the diſeaſe. They are the conſequences of pain, ſtimulus and irritation; acting on delicate and ſenſible membranes; and will be found in every caſe of ſudden death, from any abdominal diſeaſe whatever, or from any kind of poiſon taken into the ſtomach. The pulſe in this complaint, is never hard or throbbing, as in enteritis, and blood drawn in it, never exhibits any inflammatory cruſt; nor is there any difficulty in moving the belly, when the ſtomach will retain purgatives, as there is in that diſeaſe. Much experience indeed does it require, and many diſſections of ſimilar caſes, to enable us to judge and diſtinguiſh accurately between the cauſes and effects of diſeaſe; and even between the effects of diſeaſe, and the effects of death. The diſſection proceeds no further than we have mentioned; and if it did, it is but a very ſlight judgment we could form from appearances, of the preſence or abſence of noxious acrimony in the inteſtinal contents. Chemiſtry itſelf has not yet imitated, nor can it be ſuppoſed ever to imitate the operation by which chyme is converted into com-

 pletely

pletely animalized chyle; far lefs the morbid alienations of this procefs. What life is, or what the influence it exerts on the operations of a living fyftem, or in what way it is acted on, either by ftimulants or fedatives, are all matters that feem to lie beyond the fphere of our inveftigation. We can do little more than obferve and inveftigate facts. We are pretty certain, that of all the fecreted liquors, none are more fufceptible of morbid alienations than the bile; that in a healthy ftate, it is a neceffary and important agent in the chylous procefs, but when it is altered and difeafed, there is no faying of what kinds, or to what extent, acrimonious changes may be produced on the digeftive matters.

Hence, in the cure of difeafes referable to this fource, our indications are confined to the objects of diluting and expelling what is noxious. Where the nature of this is unknown, demulcents and correctors in a proper fenfe, can have no place.

In feveral cafes, however, even this is not to be undertaken without precaution, and is to be accomplifhed only in an indirect or round-about way. The irritability of the ftomach muft be taken off, before we can introduce either diluents or purgatives

tives with any effect; and the irritation arifing from pain and fpafm, muft be allayed or mitigated in order to prevent the acceffion of inflammatory affection. Nothing, in full and ftrong habits, or where the pulfe keeps tolerably firm, and where there are no fainting fits nor coldnefs of the extremities, will conduce fo effectually to the laft purpofe, as full blood-letting. But where the circumftances are reverfed, it can do no good, and the blood is often with difficulty made to flow, from the ficknefs and faintings. In fuch circumftances, a large blifter applied over the abdomen will have much more certain effects.

For the purpofe of taking off the irritability of the ftomach, and removing the vomitings, it is feldom that, under proper managment, we are difappointed in employing opium. It is almoft needlefs to fay, that fuccefs is not to be expected, in the ordinary way of giving it by the mouth. Rubbing two or three drachms of laudanum, mixed with warm fpirits, on the ftomach, will fometimes anfwer tolerably well. But a far more certain effect is to be expected, from exhibiting it by glyfter. From 60 to 100 drops of laudanum, (according to the feverity of the difeafe, and the patient's previous habits with regard to the ufe of opium), in a fmall quantity of thin and liquid ftarch, forms a proper glyfter. It will be retained in the rectum, and feldom fails to procure a complete remiffion of the fpafms, pain, and retching. The ftomach will become fteady enough to retain purgatives in moderate but continued dofes, with mild diluent liquors, in fmall quantity at a time, until the belly be fufficiently opened; always preferring, both with refpect to form and quality, fuch as pafs the ftomach with the leaft irritation; and continuing them, till we are fure the bowels are evacuated from end to end. Glyfters, though they may be ufeful to begin and promote evacuations, have only a partial operation on the bowels, and cannot of themfelves fecure our purpofe. A return of pain and retching may occafionally take place, and require a repetition of the opiate-glyfter for their abatement, with a repetition of the purgative medicines afterwards; but in this cafe, it is neceffary to watch the ftate of the pulfe, left the continuance of irritation fhould light up inflammation; which free and timous blood-letting only can prevent.

Another reafon for our prefcribing opium is, that by its acting much more on the fentient, than upon

upon the moving power, it ſo far prevents irritation, as to allow of acrimonious matters being drawn off through the inteſtines without danger, which would ruffle and ſtimulate extremely, if a temporary reduction was not thus induced on the ſenſorial power. In other words, the ſyſtem may be kept a good deal under the influence of opium, without our loſing much of the effect of purgatives.

A repetition of the purgatives, or at leaſt attention to preſerve an open belly, will be always neceſſary for ſome time. For, to whatever cauſe we may impute the diſeaſe, not only will the aliments at the time in the bowels, be diverted from the proper chylifactive proceſs, but ſuch as are taken in during its continuance, will not undergo that proceſs perfectly; or the action of the inteſtines will be weakened, and they will require an additional ſtimulus to ſecure the proper propulſion of their contents.

We do not intend to maintain, that every caſe of this diſeaſe, as we have deſcribed it, is to be with certainty referred to irritation from acrimony generated in the firſt paſſages. The paſſage of gall-ſtones, through the biliary ducts, or of urinary concretions by the ureters, the difplacement with ftrangulation of any of the bowels, will be accompanied with fymptoms very nearly fimilar: and pain, efpecially when very acute, is not always referred with much diftinctnefs to the place of the offending caufe, even by the patient himfelf. But in all *thefe* cafes, there will be fome hardnefs or fulnefs in the pulfe; and blood drawn during the complaint, will exhibit more or lefs of an inflammatory cruft. There may be retrocedent gout, or there may be a fpafmodic or nervous affection, fuch as we fee in fome hyfteric diforders fomewhat refembling this: But in all of them, except perhaps in the cafe of the gout, of which I fay nothing, becaufe I never faw it, or in the paffage of gall-ftones and urinary calculi, we can never confider our patient as fecure, until his bowels are fully cleared; and the chief part of the cure muft confift in purging *.

Another fet of difeafes arifing in this country from depravations of bile, we meet with among infants.

---

* See Appendix No. II.

fants. In the fetus, many of the internal organs are imperfect and inactive. Until birth the animal has not yet arrived at the exercise of half its functions. An entirely new and different way of life is then entered on, with a different distribution of the circulating fluid; and an increased supply of it to most of the internal organs, in particular to the liver. Plethora, then, or an unusual determination of blood to the abdominal viscera, is a necessary consequence of this change, and precedes that which, in growing animals, takes place towards the head. All the secretions performed in this part of the body, seem to be in excess, compared with those of the adult. Hence the frequency of jaundice, of the red and yellow gum, the deep yellow or green colour, so prevalent in the stools of infants, the frequency of loosenesses, gripes, cholic pains and fluxes, with the strong tendency of all their diseases to fall upon this part of the system. Acidity in the first passages, from the nature of their aliment, irritation from teething, from abounding slime, or from worms, may give occasion to many of their complaints. But very often they have their origin from a different and more dangerous source, viz. irregularity, excess, occa-

sional

ſional obſtruction and depravations in the bilious ſecretion.

Diſorders ariſing from this ſource may be in every degree. They always become ſerious, when, with ſome vomiting or purging of highly-coloured bile, or at leaſt with more or leſs bowel irregularity, the belly becomes tumid and painful, attended with fits of crying, ſeemingly from cholic pains; with ſome interruption or irregularity in the urinary diſcharge; the bowels ſometimes looſe, at other times difficultly moved; with ſtools of a green colour, and of a broken conſiſtence, intermixed occaſionally with a white, thick and plaſtic matter, and green ſlime. If occaſional ruſhes recede, and the healthful appearance of freckling on the ſkin goes off, and if it becomes pale and white, with a livid colour about the eyes and lips; and if the child becomes unable to ſuck, moans and whines in a weakened and altered tone of voice, much danger is always to be apprehended. If the diſeaſe proceeds, the eyes become fixed and ſtaring, with the pupils dilated; and much anxiety and diſtreſs is painted on the countenance. The pulſe begins to ſink, and the extremities become cold and livid, with cold ſweats over the body. Irregular catch-

ing

ing convulſions of the muſcles, of the fingers, arms and face, come on, indicating the approach of death; and the abdomen ſwells and becomes livid, ſometimes before, and always ſoon after that event.

This is the diſeaſe called by mothers and nurſes in Scotland, the *bowel-hive*. It is a dangerous inflammatory bilious diſorder; and when not ſoon relieved, very frequently proves fatal. It is brought on by diſorders of the milk, by expoſure to cold, and living in low, cold and damp ſituations.

Every thing here depends on free and timely evacuation of the bowels, repeated as long as green, viſcid, broken, white and plaſtic matter is diſcharged. Bleeding with leeches if the child is full and ſtrong; warm bathing; and bliſtering the abdomen. In weakly children, rubbing the belly with warm ſpirits may be employed. It proves little ſtimulant in this way; and may be uſed with advantage in many of the bowel-complaints of children. No purgative anſwers better in this caſe, or is more to be depended on, than calomel: but it ought always to be remembered, that in ſome of the bowel-complaints, even of very infants, full and effectual evacuation is not to be procured, except

cept by the exhibition of purgatives in very large and repeated doſes. This may be always preſumed, when the ſtools are plaſtic and ſlimy; cauſing the cloths on which they are received, to cohere and ſtick together.

Copy of a Letter to Mr W—— Aſſiſtant-Surgeon Madras, &c.

"Sir,

"I have been favoured with yours by Enſign G——. As your letter ſhews a candid inquſitiveneſs that merits information, I ſhall be ſomewhat explicit in anſwer.

"Mr G——'s is one of theſe caſes, which occur every day in this country, and oftener than is imagined in other hot climates; not ſeldom I believe in camps, and in particular ſeaſons in Europe, when bilious diſorders prevail. But it is generally overlooked, on the ſuppoſition that fluxes are ſimple diarrhœas, ariſing from miaſmata, putrid bile or crudities, or ſomething acrimonious in the firſt paſſages; and of courſe are treated with emetics,

emetics, laxatives, antifpafmodics, and bitters. Indeed, if they were only produced by fuch fimple caufes, we might generally expect fpeedy and effectual cures, by a perfeverance in the above remedies, properly adapted.

"But on the contrary, we fee them often run on to a great length; and often of precarious iffue: and to our mortification find, that fuch treatment proves palliative only for a day. This being evidently enough the cafe, we ought naturally to conjecture, that the fource of this obftinacy muft be looked for, beyond the inteftinal canal. Such is really the fact. A deep-rooted obftruction generally fupports the difeafe, in fpite of unwearied evacuations; and all affiftance becomes only palliative till this is removed.

"A want of attention to this circumftance, allows fluxes to run on to the fecond and third ftages as they are called; but which in reality are no more than different ftages of duration and weaknefs; for the difeafe has been uniformly the fame from its commencement, viz. An obftructed liver and mefentery; but chiefly the former, with fome degree of inflammation: The flux itfelf being little more than a fymptom

of

of the diſeaſe, and the effect of diſeaſed ſecretions.

"We have ſeldom reaſon to be doubtful of this cauſe; for if we have not pain to direct us, an experienced touch will diſcover the obſtructions, the tenderneſs or enlargement of the liver. I ſay an *experienced touch;* becauſe it requires frequent practical examination, to ſatisfy one with reſpect to the different degrees of hardneſs, firmneſs and ſenſibility, that conſtitute a diſeaſe of this bowel.

"However, appearances are ſeldom ſo equivocal, as to puzzle practice in general. I venture to affirm, that the grand ſource of health and diſeaſe, is connected with the natural or diſeaſed condition of the liver; and that every chronic or lingering illneſs, ariſes in a conſiderable degree from ſome defect there. In many acute diſorders, it has alſo its ſhare. But in every kind of ſickneſs, whether local or general, that is peculiar to this country, it is material to examine it. For, no perfect cures can be made, without having a ſtrict eye to it.

"The flux he has laboured under for 15 months, might originally have been cured in as many days; and even now will give but little trouble, as he has

has ſtrength enough left to bear the operation of medicines.

"His caſe from the beginning to this time, has been an obſtructed liver; and could have been at no time effectually cured, but by mercurial deobſtruents. A ſtrict diet, exerciſe, palliative and laxative medicines, to blunt and evacuate bile diſordered in its ſecretion, when the inflammatory tendency had ceaſed, might relieve for a time; and even produce a temporary cure. But they never could reſtore him to that health, or the vivid clearneſs of countenance peculiar to health; nor even prevent the relapſes he has been ſubject to, during ſo protracted an illneſs, at ſo many different periods of which, had his feelings been queſtioned, they would have been ſufficient to have pointed out the ſource and cauſe of his diſeaſe. For I find by his own account, his caſe has been in the beginning a great deal inflammatory. At preſent, his liver is only enlarged and hard, but no pain there. His flux is accompanied with gripes and teneſmus, and his look is bloated and ſallow. His urine, too, is very high-coloured. This appearance, by the by, never fails to attend liver-diſorders of any ſtanding; though it now and then happens in nervous habits

habits, and in diseases of the bile itself. But in general, it is a material index to diseases where bile prevails.

" When obstructions of the liver exist, the first digestion goes on very imperfectly ; therefore, the first indication in this case is, to clear the bowels of phlegm, and other causes of irritation. The second, to remove the obstructions of the liver ; also to restore the lost tone of the intestines, and to strengthen the system in general.

" In recent cases where tenesmus is troublesome, castor-oil is a good purge ; it operates effectually, and discharges much gelatinous stuff, from the flexures of the duodenum and colon ; and as it enters not the blood, it creates little disturbance in the system. It is therefore in recent cases a good purge. But in his case, where the bowels have been much relaxed and weakened, rhubarb, quickened with calomel, or soluble tartar, is better to answer the first intention ; repeated once, or oftener, according to the nature and complexion of the excretions.

" Proper evacuations being made ; the second indication, of removing the obstruction of the liver, is to be answered by mercury, administered but slowly ;

ſlowly; as his complaints are of long ſtanding, and his habit much relaxed. A drachm of mercurial ointment may be rubbed into his ſide daily; and ten grains of a pill compoſed of equal parts of rhubarb and calomel may be given, one night and morning, or the following:

℞. Species aromat. gr. iv.
Vitreum Antim. cerat.
Calomel. præp. utriuſque gr. iij.
Confect. Alkermes, q. s. ad bolum, man. et vesp. ſumendum.

This is to be continued till the mercury fixes in his mouth. And by this means the obſtructions will be gradually removed; and the load of ſerous humours that flow to his guts, in their preſent relaxed and irritable ſtate, will be diverted to his mouth; whereby his bowels will gain a truce from evacuations.

"As the obſtructions remove, the urine and ſtools will grow more natural, and every ſecretion leſs diſeaſed. In theſe chronic obſtructions, the friction in the application of the mercurial ointment, is alſo not without its uſe.

"As you deſire my opinion of Opiates and Aſtringents, I ſhall give it you, from experience, in a few words.

"Opiates are dangerous medicines in fluxes, and always to be uſed with fearful caution. Early in the diſorder, where the diſeaſe is putrid or inflammatory, they ſhould be given in no ſituation. Suſpending evacuations for a night, may bring on a fatal inflammation. In chronic caſes, freedom from gripes, the ſmell and nature of the evacuations by ſtool, are the only criteria to direct their uſe; for no retentions are to be made of any thing acrimonious. In ſhort, in a climate where all the capital diſorders ariſe from putrid bile, or obſtructions, nothing muſt be ſhut up.

"As to aſtringents, they are often dangerous medicines in fluxes, and always precarious. They can be uſed with no kind of ſafety, till all kinds of obſtructions are removed, and with them every thing that is putrid and diſeaſed. In the acute caſes they have fatal effects. In the more chronic they pamper and protract the diſorder; with all its concomitants, gripes, teneſmus, &c.

"When the diſeaſe becomes a ſimple diarrhœa without gripes; or theſe originating only from wind, equal parts of Prunorum Sylveſt. and the Conſerv. Aurantior. or Confect. Cardiaca is an elegant and ſafe aſtringent. The Tinct. Caſcarillæ, cold

cold bathing, and exercise, recover the conftitution from relaxation.

" Having made thefe remarks on opiates and aftringents, I come next to the fecond indication in the cafe of Mr G——; the obftruction of his liver being removed, and the other complaints abated, it is to be anfwered by mild bitters of the leaft aftringent kind. Bark, which in moft cafes of weaknefs and irritation, is an invaluable medicine, is in liver difeafes a poifon. The Flor. Chamæmel. Sem. Carvi, Sal Polychreft. of each ʒi., will make a couple of cups of bitter tea, to be drunk before and after noon. This with proper diet and exercife will be fufficient to reftore him,

" Captain Long, whom you may know, laboured under a diforder of the fame kind, but worfe, being complicated with much weaknefs, and the lofs in a great meafure of the ufe of his extremities. The fource and caufe of his complaint had alfo been overlooked, and he alfo had trifled on with the ufual medicines for fluxes, till he was reduced to extreme weaknefs. After reducing the obftruction of the liver by mercury, putting the patient in a proper train for the uſe of aſtringents, his cure was effectually completed, with

℞. Cons. Aurantior. ℥i.
Pulv. Cort. Per. ℥ß.
Pulv. Rad. Serpent. Virg. ʒij.
Tart. Vitriol. ʒi.
Syr. Aurant. q s. ad electuar.

Of this he took ℥ß in the day, and continued it ſome time. And every night when his excretions were not free, he took 10 grains of a pill compoſed of aloes, ſoap and calomel.

" Theſe are two inſtances of liver fluxes, which you have ſeen. I have met with numberleſs unfortunates from camps, and different parts of the country in the very ſame predicament; who have with great difficulty ſurvived this wreck of conſtitution.

" But it is impoſſible in a letter to enumerate the different varieties of complicated bilious diſorders, that practice daily preſents to obſervation. Nor can I in this way convey a proper idea of the nice and particular treatment, diſeaſes ariſing from putrid bile and obſtructions require. Different circumſtances and conſtitutions diverſify preſcription. Capital diſeaſes require the moſt circumſpect attention. Omiſſions or miſtakes are not to be re-

medied

medied by any future efforts; eſpecially where putrid bile lurks in the habit. Diſturbing it ſuddenly by evacuations, putting it in motion before it is well diluted and corrected, proves often like poiſon, ſuddenly fatal. Of this I have ſeen inſtances in men who were not at the time confined to their beds. As a ſtriking inſtance, alſo of the attention neceſſary in the moſt trifling complaints ariſing from bile, I can aſſure you, I have known what are called *trifling medicines*, preſcribed for ailments which were conſidered equally trifling, productive of very ſerious diſorders.

"For example, I have ſeen a courſe of bitters, ordered for what was imagined a windy relaxed ſtomach, produce obſtructions; and in inflammatory habits, a real inflammation of that bowel. Such accidents as theſe, awaken a man's caution. But it is a practical fact, that no ſtrong aſtringent bitter can be uſed here with impunity, unleſs the caſe is really ſimple relaxation. Mixing the gentleſt kinds with neutral ſalts is only ſafe. Indeed, it is perhaps a problem in phyſic, how long the uſe of aſtringents may be continued with ſafety, or without danger of inducing ſome other diſorder.

" Before I conclude this letter, though ſomewhat foreign to the ſubject of yours, I cannot avoid putting you on your guard againſt a diſorder of the liver, which, from its being overlooked, I have once ſeen in Europe, and ſeveral times here, attended with fatal conſequences. The complaint I mean, is what is called the *liver-cough*. The obſtruction in this caſe, is pretty generally accompanied with ſome degree of inflammation and pain; though ſeldom acute, unleſs preſſed with the fingers; or when the external membrane is alſo affected. But it often happens without pain or inflammation. The cough is entirely a ſymptomatic complaint, and is the miſleading ſymptom of the diſeaſe.

" The patient pronounces his own caſe a cold, and is put on a courſe of ineffectual pectorals, takes exerciſe, and ſhifts his ſituation for health, until his liver either ſuppurates, or becomes a maſs of irrecoverable obſtructions. In every irritable or inflammatory habit, any miſtake at the commencement of the diſeaſe, is of the moſt dangerous conſequence. The liver, diaphragm and lungs, adhere and ſuppurate. A purulent ſpitting ſucceeds; and inſtead of a pure uniform pus, the ſubſtance of the liver

liver is expectorated with a deep hollow cough; in form of glandular membranes, of a purplish bloody parenchymatous look. This disease, like all other inflammations of the liver, is very tractable in the beginning by evacuations, relaxing antiphlogistic medicines and mercury.

"Such cases as the above I have met with, and have been happy enough to effect some cures even in this advanced stage.

"It is to be observed, in all disorders of the lungs of any standing, the liver is always affected; but in this case the lungs are but secondarily so, and never give any trouble, if the obstruction of the liver is removed.

"In them there are neither tubercles nor infarctions. The breathing, except in inflammatory cases, is never affected, and the symptomatic complaint of cough and pain in the shoulder, may always be mitigated by lying on the back, with the head low, and the legs raised.

"To the above I shall add another disorder, which is entirely of the liver kind.

"Agues are by no means frequent in the dry sandy soil of this coast; but quotidian remittents often happen here, from inflammatory obstruction of the liver. I ſay *remittents*, becauſe the fever never goes entirely off; though the quotidian ague fits are very regular in their attacks. The patient in ſuch caſes tells you only he has got the fever and ague, with a pain at the pit of his ſtomach. But his report is not to be truſted without farther examination; both in the ſtanding and lying poſture. On preſſing with your fingers towards his right ſide, he will complain of much pain and tenderneſs; and his urine will be very high coloured. Sometimes he will have a pain in his right ſhoulder; and generally he has a liver cough. This is a complicated caſe; though there is in reality no contra-indications in the cure of it. The inflammation and obſtruction of the liver, are the proximate cauſe of the diſeaſe; and all its different ſymptoms. Veneſection is immediately neceſſary; and if the ſtomach ſeems loaded, an emetic may ſafely be adminiſtered after it; but it ſhould be ſuch as will operate eaſily, and open the belly. Such I found the following in all bilious caſes:

Vin. Ipecac. et Antimon. utriuſque ℥ ſs.

Oxym. Scillit. ʒ vi. M.

"Notwithſtanding the continued fever, a drachm of mercurial ointment may be rubbed into the ſide, morning

morning and evening, after fomenting it. Saline draughts with nitre, or tartar emetic, ought to be given every three or four hours; and the bleeding repeated if neceſſary. The ague and cough require no attention. They will diminiſh as the mercury takes effect; and entirely ceaſe when a ſpitting comes on. Any bilious attacks that happen during the interval, are to be relieved by emetics, caſtor oil, or ſoluble tartar and glyſters, as circumſtances may require. We meet here with quotidians of two years ſtanding, attended with a very irregular ſtate of the bowels, and on every acceſſion of the fit, ſuch an aſtoniſhing ſecretion of bile as to produce a real cholera morbus.

"On the ſubject of agues I ſhall obſerve to you, that bark is ſeldom neceſſary in the cure of them; and often unſafe; except in caſes of great weakneſs and relaxation, or where the nervous ſyſtem is much affected. On the contrary, evacuants, neutral ſalts, and deobſtruents are ſeldom ineffectual. However, where the indications are not ſufficiently marked, and where difficulty ariſes about the propriety of exhibiting particular medicines, the following criteria, with reſtrictions, may ſerve as a guide.

"When

" When bark does not ſucceed in ſtopping the fits, and preventing relapſes ; deobſtruents, neutral ſalts, and relaxing medicines, with evacuants, according to circumſtances, are more likely to anſwer. But whether in agues, or in diſeaſes induced by obſtructions of the viſcera, if the urine is high coloured in the intervals of the fit, or during the courſe of the diſeaſe, aſtringents of every kind are to be avoided, as infinite miſchief may be done by them, eſpecially if the diatheſis be inflammatory, or if putrid bile lurks in the primæ viæ ; from which often ariſes wonderful and aſtoniſhing effects in the ſyſtem. Sudden fevers are lighted up, and all the variety of nervous affection ; according to the degree of its acrimony, and the peculiar idioſyncraſy of the patient.

" The caſe of a gentleman who was under my care not many days ago, will exemplify this. He was young, healthy and florid, when he was ſuddenly taken ill with fever, dry ſkin, and his tongue as white as a ſheet ; his urine like porter, with a highly alkaline ſmell. Great heat and fulneſs about the præcordia. Pulſe ſometimes high, ſometimes low, but always as quick as poſſible. Great reſtleſſneſs and agitation of his whole frame. Sometimes

times the deepeſt dejection of ſpirits, even to crying; ſometimes raving, horrors and general ſpaſms. Sometimes crying for wine to ſupport him. Sometimes crying for water to allay an unquenchable thirſt. All theſe tranſitions were diſplayed during my firſt viſit, which happened in a few hours after his being firſt ſeized.

"This appears clear enough to be a caſe of putrid bile, operating in the ſyſtem; and is one of thoſe caſes, where the patient is either out of danger, or extinguiſhed in a few hours.

"The whole indication of cure in ſuch caſes is, to dilute and evacuate the irritating cauſe; by attemperating medicines, to quiet the diſturbance in the ſyſtem occaſioned by it.

"Stimulants have no place here, notwithſtanding the variety of nervous affections. They unavoidably aggravate every ſymptom. Emetics ruffle too much to be ventured on, when the whole ſyſtem is diſordered; beſides the danger of their ſetting in motion at once, a deluge of putrid bile, which is never done without inſtant riſk.

"For this gentleman I ordered a purging glyſter immediately; and his legs to be fomented in ſalt and water; till a ſolution of one ounce of manna,

and

and half an ounce of ſoluble tartar, in twelve ounces of water, could be ſent him.

"Of this he was directed to take four table ſpoonfuls every hour, till it ſhould operate four times; which brought away ſome frothy bile of an intolerable ſtench, like the workings of a beer caſk in its appearance. This was far from being ſufficient to produce any conſiderable effect. He was however ſenſibly relieved, and it was no ſmall ſatisfaction, from the nature of the excretions, to find the diſeaſe in my power. As ſoon as the effect of the laxative was over, I directed him to take every three hours, a table-ſpoonful of the following:

℞. Camphoræ gr. x.
Mucil. Gum. Arabic. ℥i.
Amygdal. dulc. decort. ij.
Terantur optimè ſimul, et adde
Jalap. Salin. ℥ x.
Tart. Emetic. gr. j.
Syr. Sach. ℥ij. M.

This to be continued in the intervals of purging and to uſe clear Rheniſh whey as common drink. He paſſed a more tolerable night, leſs reſtleſs, leſs oppreſſed, and his head leſs affected. The day following

following he was indeed worſe. Another and more active purge was preſcribed, compoſed of

Fol. Sennæ ʒj.
Mannæ ℥ij.
Tart. Solubil. ʒiij.
Sem. Carvi ʒß.

Infuſed in eight ounces of boiling water, one half to be taken early in the morning, and the other two hours after.

This operated five times. The ſtools were of the ſame nature and ſmell, but plentiful, and every ſymptom abated conſiderably. After the operation of this purge, his urine and tongue remained the ſame; but he was much more compoſed, with fewer ſpaſms, and fewer attacks of the depreſſion of ſpirits. His ſkin was moiſter, and his pulſe regular and leſs frequent.

"It only remained now to prepare the remainder of the bile for expulſion. He was therefore directed to drink frequently, and take his medicines regularly for a couple of days; and the third day in the morning, the ſame purge was repeated, with the addition of half a drachm more of ſenna. This operated very effectually, and brought away much gelatinous ſtuff and bile; and the evening of that day his urine became natural and clear.

clear. His complaints all vaniſhed, though his tongue was but little altered. Nothing further was neceſſary, but to leave a purge with him, to continue the Rheniſh whey, and to uſe light diet until he recovered more ſtrength. But as theſe diſorders, with many others of the putrid bilious kind originate in the liver, relapſes cannot be prevented, nor perfect recoveries made, without removing every obſtruction, and reſtoring the ſecretions to health. For though all acrimonious and putrid accumulations, ariſing from diſeaſed ſecretions, are removed by well-timed evacuations; yet indigeſtion and frequent collections may ſoon occaſion the ſame ſcene to be acted over again, if obſtructions are not removed, and healthy bile reſtored to perform Nature's firſt and greateſt operation in the animal economy. We therefore ſhould never think it ſufficient to ſave the patient from immediate and preſent danger. It is incumbent on us alſo to remove the latent defect, which is the principal ſource of all; the obſtructed ſtate of the liver and meſenteric glands. The excretions and urine are minutely to be attended to; and as circumſtances require, gentler or ſtronger mercurial deobſtruents, with mild bitters and neutral

tral ſalts, with occaſional vacuants, are to be exhibited; and ſtrict diet is to be recommended, till the health and conſtitution be perfectly reſtored; otherwiſe our ſervices are flattering rather than uſeful,—if I may be allowed the compariſon, like the ſplendid actions of the General, which often acquire to him reputation and honour, but are productive of no real advantage to the State.

" I could furniſh you with a variety of ſuch caſes, and a multitude of ſuch hiſtories, of other complicated bilious diſorders which came daily under my notice, but they would ſwell this letter to a volume, though it already exceeds the bounds I had preſcribed to it. I ſhall therefore only further obſerve to you in general, That bile, in different ſtates and conditions, produces the appearance, and apes almoſt every other diſorder, and of conſequence, much attention and experience are required, to diſtinguiſh properly its operation and effects. In this country there are but few ſimple fluxes, ſimple agues, or coughs, or indeed ſimple diſorders. And you may be aſſured, that when the liver and primæ viæ are not conſidered as the grand ſources of diſeaſe, continual and ſerious blunders will be committed. Mercury, in judicious hands,

hands, is a ſafe and tractable medicine; and as it is the only powerful and effectual deobſtruent in glandular obſtructions, it is of conſequence the only medicine that can be depended on, in the latent defects of the ſyſtem, which entail diſeaſes or impede recovery. However, it often requires aſſiſtance from other medicines; ſuch as are antiſpaſmodic or aqueous to waſh the glands, and increaſe the ſecretions in general. And it alſo requires aſſiſtance adapted to the effects the diſeaſe has produced on the conſtitution. For example, in venereal and other habits, where the ſolids are much relaxed, the blood poor and flimſy, mercury without bark will ſpread every ulcer, induce fibrillæ, and increaſe every ſymptom. In acute diſeaſes, evacuations, neutral ſalts, and relaxing medicines, render it ſafe and effectual. In irritable habits it requires management, as its operation is chiefly on the ſolids. But the idea of its injuring the conſtitution, by deſtroying the craſis of the blood, is without foundation. On the contrary, it is but too apt to leave behind it an inflammatory diatheſis: So much ſo indeed, that I would recommend to you a general rule in all ſevere attacks of diſeaſe, where mercury has preceded, to bleed

bleed early and freely. For, watching, fatigues, and bodily exerciſe of the ſevereſt kinds, have not greater effects in waſting the thinner parts of the blood, and producing a denſity of it, than mercurial courſes. The mild air of this country is very favourable to the operation of mercury, and there are many diſeaſes here, for which it is infallible, with fair play and judicious management.

" You may obſerve, I have been ſomewhat general on my anſwer to yours. But I was willing to throw into it as much information as the compaſs of a letter would admit of. Upon the whole, it contains a few remarks which you may improve to your advantage. To have been circumſtantially minute was impoſſible, it being rather a ſubject for a whole volume, than for a few ſheets. Hoſpitals and practice can only realize theſe hints; and if I can at any time render you any aſſiſtance, I ſhall be ready to do it.

I am, Dear Sir, &c.

J. PAISLEY.

" P. S. I have added the ſtate of our hoſpital (Military) at Madras *, to ſhew you the prevailing diſeaſes along the coaſt for this month.

Venereals, - - -	50
Quotidian remittents, - -	2
Simple bilious fevers, - -	30
Bilious fevers, with viſceral obſtructions,	15
Simple fluxes, - -	20
Liver fluxes, and fluxes from viſceral obſtruction, - -	98
Chronic viſceral obſtruction from impaired habit, - -	69

---

* See Appendix, No. III.

ULCERS

ULCERS

AND

HOSPITAL SORES.

THE Naval Hoſpital at Madras, conſiſted of a large ſquare of building; or rather of a ſhade of one ſtory, open every where on the inner ſide; and within a few hundred yards of the ſea beach, detached from all other houſes. A ſhade open on all ſides was conſtructed within the ſquare, and extending its whole length, for the accommodation of patients with wounds, ulcers, and ſores. And ſuch was the freedom of ventilation through the whole, that no bad or ſickly ſmell was ever perceived, except cloſe to ſome bad putrid ulcer, or patient with a putrid flux. The cheapneſs of labour, and the liberality of the gentlemen who had the contract, provided us with servants for sweeping, washing, and all the purposes of cleanliness, to our utmost wish. Ventilation was our only concern; for warmth or shelter we needed to have no care. Under circumstances so favourable, we were led to impute the general intractability of our ulcers and sores, rather to the influence of other causes, than to the fault of foul and contaminated hospital air;—either to the effect of local circumstances; the state and situation of the settlement, and of the town of Madras; or to the state of the air and constitution of the climate, inducing a weakened and relaxed condition of the extreme vessels, (probably in many instances combined with a latent scorbutic taint), which rendered the healing of all sores, or the separation of the dead, and renovation of new and living parts, an uncommonly tedious and difficult process. A peculiar degree of acrimony in the matter of sores and ulcers, was also very remarkable, and presented an additional obstacle; and made it very difficult to maintain the proper condition in their vessels, for accomplishing the healing process.

That the influence of the climate, and state of the air, was sometimes connected with these depravations,

pravations, we had undoubted proof at the ſetting in of the north-eaſt monſoon, on the 14th October 1782, when almoſt every ſtump, ſore, and ulcer in the hoſpital, got foul, and put on a bad appearance; while in the cool and dry weather that ſucceeded about the middle of November, and during the month of December, thoſe all got better; and more of them were healed up within the laſt month, than ever happened during any other period. Similar changes were obſerved to take place on other occaſions, when the alteration in the ſtate of the weather was not at all remarkable; but never to any thing near the ſame degree as in this. That a taint of ſea-ſcurvy in the blood, ſometimes contributed its ſhare to the degeneracy and ill condition of our ſores, we had good evidence in the appearance of the ſore itſelf, even when ſcarcely any marks of it could be otherwiſe detected in the habit.

For, in many caſes, from ſhips newly arrived from England, or from long cruiſes in the India ſeas, the appearance which this taint never fails to communicate to ſores or ulcers, was evidently perceivable;—an ulcer with thick and livid edges, and a ſuffuſed dun or yellow colour, ſpreading ſome way round it, readily diſpoſed to bleed upon the ſlighteſt preſſure; or, inſtead of purulent matter, a bloody ſerum oozing out; or the parts ſwelled up, and the ſore covered with a hard and firm coagulum of a red colour, compoſing a kind of membranous cruſt, raiſed high above its ſurface. Theſe appearances are always deciſive of true ſea-ſcurvy. But they are not always ſo diſtinctly marked as to attract our attention. An ulcer with livid edges, and a yellow broad margin, with a diſchage partly ſanious, partly purulent, and a tendency to bleed on friction, marks alſo pretty certainly ſome degree of the ſame taint. We found much more difficulty in correcting this diatheſis at Madras, than uſually happens, where vegetable, or even farinaceous diet can be procured in any tolerable plenty.

The air of a large hoſpital might contribute ſomewhat to the production of this taint; but I am perſuaded, the local ſituation of the town, and ſtate of the ſettlement at that period, had a very conſiderable ſhare. The country round was more than once overrun, and plundered by the horſe troops of Hyder Ally. So that our ſupply, even of freſh meat, and much more of vegetables and fruits,

fruits, was by far too ſcanty. And a few imperfectly cultivated and unripened fruits, with the cocoa-nut juice called *toady*, was all we could procure for our ſcorbutics. Another ſource of unhealthineſs ariſes from the ſituation of the town, and fort of Madras itſelf, built upon a low, flat and ſandy beach, and ſurrounded almoſt entirely with ſtagnant ſwamps, or ponds of ſtagnant water, which are not only a receptacle for every ſort of corruption and filth, but have their edges, as well as the beach on the other ſide, covered at all hours of the day with the natives, in the act of relieving nature from her burdens, to take advantage of the water for waſhing afterwards, which is their invariable cuſtom. What a ſource of putrid exhalations under a vertical ſun! The ſtreets, lanes and alleys, formed only of beaten ſand, admitted of no ſweeping or cleaning: Nor did there ſeem to exiſt while we were there, any ſort of police for that purpoſe; or for removing nuiſances of any kind. So that if it had not been for the number of *Brammany* kites, carion crows, and *parriar* dogs, together with an innumerable multitude of large flies, all conſtantly employed in the office of ſcavengers, in removing this offenſive maſs, Madras, in my opinion, could not have been habitable. How much better regulated ſuch things may be now, I know not.

Famine was alſo at this period ſpreading ſickneſs and death. The miſerable natives were daily falling down, or laying themſelves down, an eaſy and unreſiſting prey to it, in every ſtreet, ſtall and lane about Black Town. Nor did anybody ſeem to take any further concern with them, than to carry them off, and throw them down at the back of the *bound hedge*, (a kind of ditch and bank planted with bamboos, which had ſerved to mark out the boundaries of the firſt European ſettlements in India,) converted literally at this period into a real Golgotha, the place of many a human bone and ſkull.

At this time the country was frequently overrun by Hyder Ally's *Louties*, or irregular horſe-troops; and great numbers of the inhabitants, after being plundered, or having their property deſtroyed, were driven to ſeek refuge within the walls of Madras. A great number of the rice-ſhips had been loſt in the monſoon. And the Engliſh fleet having ſailed to Bombay for repairs, the Bay of

Bengal

Bengal was left open to the operations of the French, with no other protection to the rice-ſhips from that quarter, (upon which Madras depends for a great part of its ſupplies,) than the ſpirited and active exertions of Captain Gower, in the Medea frigate, could afford them. The conſequence was, an extraordinary riſe in the price of rice. The company uſed ſome meaſures to relieve the general diſtreſs. Once or twice a week, a *Peon*, or *De-baſh* or ſome company's ſervant, under ſome ſuch gibberiſh name, ſet out from the fort, making a kind of hallowing noiſe, whereby he gathered all the beggars about him, and from an apron or ſaſh, full of *fenams*, (a ſmall ſilver coin of about 2½d.), diſtributed as long as he could maintain his feet among the crowd, to every hand that was held out. When he was in danger of being trodden down or overturned, he broke from them, ran to a certain diſtance, and began again the ſame diſtribution, without minding who were the followers, or who they were that received, ſo as he gave to every hand a piece, leaving the ſtronger to rob and plunder the weaker as they thought fit. Whether any thing more effectual was done

done I was ignorant, but this I ſaw again and again.

Another appearance in our hoſpital ulcers, and which I had obſerved in ſhips in India, before attending at the hoſpital; and which I thought owing to ſimple relaxation of fibre, particularly affecting the vaſcular ſyſtem, was a diſcharge of a vaſt quantity of matter upon the ſurface of the ſores, of a conſiſtence altogether differing from pus, and reſembling exactly gluten, or what is called *inflammatory buff* on the furface of blood; of a conſiſtence ſo ſtrongly adherent and elaſtic, as not to be wiped off, but with the utmoſt difficulty. This is to be met with moſt frequently in ulcers of the toes and feet, often after amputation of the toes; and while this kind of diſcharge laſts, the ſore never ſuffers any change for the worſe; but neither does it contract or heal, nor do any ſort of applications produce any change, except aſtringents. If theſe were applied with this matter on the ſurface, they only converted it into a firm tough cruſt, without affecting at all the veſſels of the ſore. Poultices made ſoft with oil, and applied cold, had moſt effect in diſolving this, ſo that the ſore could be wiped clean, and then ſolutions of blue vitriol, or, or, what perhaps did ftill better, the application of plain fpirits on a bit of charpee, foon contracted the veffels, fo as to prevent more of the glutinous part of the blood, than could be converted into good pus, from being thrown out upon it. And the cicatrization generally proceeded readily when this impediment was removed.

Some reafonable explanation could thus be made of thefe feveral appearances and conditions of our fores. But there were others of a different and more important kind, for which it was not fo eafy to account.

Inftead of the cellular membrane and foft parts being principally affected, the difeafe much more frequently occupied the hard and folid parts; the bones, tendons and periofteum. This in many inftances might be owing to previous hurts and bruifes, which affect more the hard parts, but very often nothing of this kind could be traced. Sometimes there appeared only a fmall and fuperficial ulcer, covered over with a tough gelatinous matter, with the bottom parts fwelled and puffed up; and when we got the fore in fome meafure clean, we found the tendons, where any were in the way, either fwelled up, or bare and dead in many places;

places; ſo that they rotted away to a great length beyond the extent of the ſore; or it was found neceſſary to cut them through, and very often we found matter confined below them. If a bone was near, it was uniformly found bare, or at leaſt the perioſteum ſloughy and diſeaſed to a great extent. And this we ſometimes found, where there appeared only a ſuperficial ulcer of no great ſize, ſeeming to extend no deeper that the cellular membrane, looking clean and granulating, and without ſinuſes. The diſeaſe appeared to have begun in the perioſteum, and to have extended outwards. Whenever, therefore, we found an ulcer with the bottom parts puffed up, or higher than the neighbouring ſurface, we made ourſelves ſure, though it looked clean, there was miſchief below. Indeed, every healing ulcer ought to be attended with contraction and ſinking of the parts affected, and if it is otherwiſe, ſomething wrong is always to be ſuſpected.

In many caſes, where the ulcer was ſituated in the middle of a limb, eſpecially the leg; if it was of any conſiderable ſize, with the bone expoſed and carious, we very generally found the perioſteum diſeaſed, or ſeparated and deſtroyed, to a much larger

larger extent, than either the dimenſions of the external ulcer, or the extent of the caries of the bone. Even where the edges of the ulcer ſeemed adhering to the bone all round, on trying with a probe, theſe were eaſily ſeparated, and the perioſteum was found wanting.

Exfoliation of diſeaſed bone, again, was commonly a difficult and imperfect proceſs in this country. Inſtead of caſting off in one piece, the bone came away in ſmall ſpongy carious worm-eaten like bits, while fleſhy granulations ſpringing up from the ſubſtance where bone had come off, and theſe inoſculating with ſimilar granulations from the edges of the ſore, when a new piece of bone looſened and came away, a ſloughy diſeaſed ſtate of the adjoining parts was occaſioned; and this was renewed as often as there were any parts of the diſeaſed bone to come off. We ſeldom had occaſion to know in what manner ſores of this kind could heal up; or whether ſound and healthy bone could have been formed out of theſe fleſhy granulations: For in moſt caſes, if the ulcer was of any conſiderable ſize, or was near the end of a bone or any of the large joints, and the deſtruction of the perioſteum was of large extent, (and theſe were

moſt

moſt commonly the conditions), it became abſolutely neceſſary to have recourſe to amputation at laſt. The diſeaſe of the bone came always to reach as far, or farther, than the diſeaſe of its membrane, and ſooner or later, the external ulcer followed the ſame courſe. Hectic fever was the certain conſequence, and proved as certainly fatal, if the member was not removed. Something ſimilar ſometimes happened after amputation, and occaſioned long ſtanding and troubleſome ulcerations and exfoliations, even in caſes where every thing favourable to the healing of the ſtump might have been reckoned on; even where the bone had been very well covered at the time of the operation, and ſcarcely expoſed to the external air at all. In ſome caſes, this happened after the ſtump had been perfectly healed up, and the patient had been uſing his wooden leg. A remarkable inſtance of this was in the caſe of *Henry Arthur*, whoſe leg had been taken off above the knee, whether on board ſhip, or at the hoſpital, I did not know, he being already a patient in the hoſpital when I came to attend. It was indeed a pyramidical ſtump, but it had been healed up above 12 months; and the man had long uſed his wooden leg. Small ulcerations

ulcerations and collections of matter formed in ſeveral places about the cicatrix. On the firſt examination with the probe, the inſtrument could be paſſed its whole length all round, and within the middle of the bone, which was every where denuded of the perioſteum. The diſcharge was ichorous and offenſive, and ſoon became intolerably fetid; tinging the probe of a hepar-ſulphur colour, every time it was introduced. The bone began at laſt to looſen, and by degrees puſhed outwards, till it came away by a kind of exfoliation, which was almoſt ſingular with us, viz. in one entire piece, from the trochanter minor, nearly nine inches in length. The external ſurface of the bone was ſmooth and little corroded, but within, the cancelli and inner tables were much deſtroyed; in ſo much, that the whole reſembled nearly the middle piece of a flute. Little more was required for this caſe, than to ſupport the ſtrength by wine, bark and nouriſhing diet, and to waſh out the parts frequently, with decoction of bark, and tincture of myrrh. There was no occaſion for any dilatations, the ulcerations having ſufficiently opened up the cicatrix at an early period. About four months after the bone came away, the openings were nearly ly healed up, and the whole thigh felt almoſt as hard and firm as the other. I could not prevail with him to allow me to retain the ſeparated bone; his intention being to exhibit it, with a view to an augmentation of his ſmart-money at the Cheſt of Chatham, for which the neceſſary certificates were furniſhed him.

Our large ulcers at the hoſpital were always much diſpoſed, when they got foul, to put on a gangrenous appearance. This for the moſt part was only a local affection, ariſing from a peculiar acrimony of the diſcharge, occaſioned by relaxation and torpor of circulation in the extreme veſſels. It was by far moſt frequent in ulcers of the legs, toes and feet. The edges of the ſore would get inflamed, become black, and ſlough off by little and little, with a half ſanious diſcharge, till the ſore became greatly enlarged in its whole circumference, while the reſt perhaps kept clean, and diſcharged good pus, with healthy-looking granulations. This was in general ſoon corrected by antiſeptic lotions; and the application of pledgets dipped in them, ſuch as Decoct. Cort. Peruv. and Flor. Chamæmel. with Tinct. Myrrh., poultices, wine, and meat diet, provided the conſtitution was tolerably

tolerably ſound. But very often the ſore would become ſloughy and get black all over. The circulation ſtopped in its veſſels; and a thin black ſanies came to be poured out from the half-living parts; with the edges livid and inflamed ſome way round, without any ſeparation or caſting off of the dead parts by all the means we could uſe. In this ſtate the ſore would often continue for many days, until hectic fever came on, from the abſorption of putrid matter, and deſtroyed the patient. Many ulcers that were at firſt ſuperficial, and free of ſinuſes, without any perceptible cauſe took this courſe; or were prevented for a long period from healing by this diſpoſition. Very ſeldom had we any ſphacelated limbs, with general ſwelling, inflammation, redneſs and tumour of the whole member, exanthematous and yellow ſuffuſions, ſuch as are to be met with from violent contuſions in other countries; except in a few inſtances among the wounded, after actions, eſpecially the ſanguine and robuſt, who had but newly arrived from England. Nothing like true phlegmon or phlegmonic inflammation appeared at the hoſpital; and any thing of the nature of eryſipelas was unknown there.

P We

We always had a great number of ill-conditioned gangrenous ulcers, or ulcers with gangrenous inflammation, confined to the edges of the fore only; fometimes fpreading, fometimes ftationary, or alternating with a clean furface and healthy granulations, for a long period of time. The leaft neglect or lodgment of matter, or inattention to cleanlinefs in dreffing, very readily brought on fuch a gangrenous condition in fores. The matter foon became fo acrid, as to tinge the probe of a fhining brown colour, and to produce corrofion and fphacelus.

Bark did fo little good in thefe fort of cafes, that we laid it afide altogether. I was doubtful, whether in India it ever bettered the condition of any fore. In two cafes of ulcers of this fort in the foot, opium feemed to have a good effect in ftopping the courfe of gangrene; but in many of the larger fores it produced no effect at all. Camphor was tried internally, and did good in feveral inftances.

GENERAL

GENERAL TREATMENT.

We have mentioned, that the correction of ſcorbutic diatheſis, which may be ſuppoſed to have had a very general influence upon the condition of our ulcers, was a matter of more difficulty at Madras, than uſually happens in other ſituations. Wherever this influence was diſtinguiſhable from the appearance of the ſore, or the known ſituation of the patient previous to the complaint; the aſſiſtance of internal correctors, as far as we could command them, was not overlooked, eſpecially at the firſt outſet. Wine, vegetables, and ſuch fruits as we could procure, were given freely; and I obſerved, that wherever, under ſuch circumſtances, ſores were diſpoſed to bleed eaſily, a doze of elixir of vitriol in a large draught of water, twice a-day, was of much ſervice in checking this.

In all contuſed wounds, if it be a matter of much conſequence in colder climates, on the firſt formation of ſinuſes, or lodgment of matter, to lay them open, and give the matter free vent, it is doubly ſo in this, where every thing ſtagnant in the ſyſtem, runs with ſuch rapidity into a ſtate of

 putreſcent

putrefcent and gangrenous acrimony. But this behoved to be done early or not at all; for after finufes had been formed, and lodgments of matter eftablifhed, and the edges or furface of the fore had begun to become black and gangrenous; the more we fcarified and dilated, the more need there appeared for thefe operations. Scarification in fuch circumftances, only carried the acrid matter deeper, and extended the mifchief. In fhort, nothing of this kind was ever attended with advantage, but while the fore or ulcer was in a tolerable healthy ftate, and the difcharge not yet become fanious and brown. Whenever tendons came in the way, and appeared foft and fpongy, of a dead white colour, and fwelled up, we were fure that matter was confined below them, or among their fheaths; and that they would never recover to a found ftate. So that, let the importance, or confequence of the tendon be what it might, we found it the beft way to cut it through, and remove as much of it as was difeafed, at once. Tendinous aponeurofes of mufcles behoved to be treated in the fame manner. Purulent matter was often confined by them, and as they were generally long of giving

giving way, it was thought moſt adviſable to divide them with the knife.

Whenever a large ulcer came to affect the parts near any of the large joints; if the bone was carious, and the perioſteum ſeparated and diſeaſed, beyond the diſeaſed portion of the bone; we were always forced to amputate at laſt, on account of hectic fever, the imperfect exfoliation of the bones, and the ſpreading of the ulcer from this cauſe, as well as from a bad diſpoſition in the blood, or of its own veſſels. Out of fifteen caſes of amputation, of the large limbs for ulcers of this ſort in the year 1782, we loſt only four, and I am perſuaded more of theſe might have been ſaved, if recourſe had been had to it ſooner; for none of the patients were loſt by any conſequences that aroſe from the operation, but ſunk under the hectic fever which had come on before it was done. Some patients alſo with ſpreading gangrenous ſores of the legs and feet, were probably loſt from an idea that was entertained, that gangrene and mortification depends always on a diſeaſe of the ſyſtem, and on a morbid condition of the ſolids and fluids, which muſt be corrected before any operation can ſucceed; and it muſt be confeſſed, that the directions in books of ſurgery, generally run in this way; at leaſt they commonly direct, that we ſhould wait till nature makes an attempt to ſeparate the dead from the living parts. But this opinion, ſo far at leaſt as affects Indian practice, and the *hoſpital gangrene* of that country, is not well founded; nor perhaps with reſpect to ſuch mortification as is the immediate conſequence of external injury in general *.

A caſe that occurred in the Medea frigate on her return to England, may here be put down, though

* The following inſtance fell under my knowledge. A young man in conſequence of fracture and tight bandaging of the fore-arm by a country bone-ſetter in the ſouth of Scotland, had a mortification brought on it. The ſurgeon who was called, found it advanced above the elbow, and proceeding ſo rapidly, as to make it doubtful, whether it might not reach the ſhoulder before his amputating inſtruments could be brought him from Dumfries, a diſtance of ſeven miles. They were but juſt got in time, and the arm was taken off within two inches of the head of the humerus, and very near to the diſcoloured part of the ſkin. After the amputation, every thing ſucceeded perfectly, and the ſtump healed very quickly.

though no certain or unequivocal inferences can be drawn from it. The ſhip was diſmaſted in a gale of wind off the Azores. Among a number of men hurt and wounded by the fall of the maſts, we had one with a fracture of the thigh bone, which did well; and another with fracture of the tibia and fibula near the ankle joint; ſimple it was indeed, but the bones broken into ſeveral pieces. Fractured limbs are unhappy caſes to manage in a gale of wind; and this gale laſted for many days. Though in the laſt caſe there was no tight bandaging, the leg began to mortify about the fractured parts, and ſwelled much. By the time we got our diſabled ſhip to anchor under the lee of St Michael, the ſwelling had reached the thigh; and ecchymoſis had extended on one ſide ſome-way above the knee. The man had alſo received a large wound upon the outſide of the fore-arm, whereby the fleſh and muſcles were torn off from the bone, about half of the length; but this had begun to digeſt, and was looking well. The poor fellow was very willing to have his leg taken off, and this was done a little way above the knee, with ſome difficulty, on account of the great ſwelling; and ſo near to the ecchymoſis on the ſkin, that a ſmall portion of it was at one place left above the circular inciſion. For three days he did very well, and the fever and quickneſs of pulſe which he had before, was in a great meaſure gone off. On the fourth he complained of ſome pain of his belly, and that he could not paſs his urine. Having had no ſtool from the time of the operation, a doſe of caſtor-oil was given him; ſoon after which he fell into convulſive fits, and he died in leſs than an hour. On inſpecting the ſtump immediately after death, the ſwelling of the thigh was ſo much reduced, as to looſen all the bandages. A fine ſuppuration was beginning to appear, and the ſkin laid over it was adhering. The ecchymoſis left above the inciſion at one ſpot, as formerly mentioned, was now quite gone off, and the ſkin had returned to its natural colour.

It may be proper to remark, what every naval ſurgeon will be aware of, that this caſe could not have fair play. The patient's habit was full, and would have required plentiful bleeding, laxatives or glyſters, &c. From the ſtate of the weather, none of theſe could be employed.

In

In the gangrenous and ſphacelated ulcers at the hoſpital, it was with much regret, I ſaw many ſink under hectic fever from the abſorption, before the diſcharge could be corrected ; and that in many caſes, this was not to brought about by all our remedies. It was a hard caſe to take off limbs on account of ulcers of no great extent, and which might have been cured without difficulty in other ſituations. But the alternative had been ſo often fatal, that we were forced at laſt to have recourſe to it. It was firſt tried in the caſe of *John Gibſon*, a fine young lad of 20. He was ſent to the hoſpital with an ulcer on the back-part of the leg, where the gaſtrocnemius muſcle begins to grow tendinous. It was of no great extent, and appeared to be only ſuperficial, but the ſurface was black, and the diſcharge thin and ichorous. The edges were livid and inflamed ſome way round ; yet there was but little ſwelling of the leg. It remained in this ſtate for five or ſix days, unchanged by all the applications we could deviſe. It did not ſpread, but penetrated deeper among the fibres of the internal muſcle, diſcharging a great deal of thin black ſanious fluid ; and a conſiderable degree of heat, thirſt, and quickneſs of pulſe had come

on.

on. The leg was taken off about mid-day; and by ten at night, the heat, thirft, and quicknefs of pulfe had entirely gone off. The ftump looked well at the firft dreffing, and was foon healed up, without any untoward fymptom. How far this practice was followed afterwards, the notes I had taken do not exprefs, farther than that it was adopted to the faving of fome lives; and from recollection, I am prety certain it was followed in fimilar cafes, and that any difappointments, or ill confequences, if they had followed, would have been recorded.

In other countries, inflammation, when it affects tendinous or membranous parts, generally runs high; and though they fuppurate unkindly and with difficulty, this is always attended with much inflammation and pain. But here it was quite otherwife, the inflammation never ran high enough, and it terminated moft commonly in gangrene; efpecially in cafes where the toes and feet were affected. Whenever an ulcer fo fituated, got fo deep as to affect the aponeurofes, fheaths and tendons, it was very apt to get foul and gangrenous; and the matter was ready to fpread and infinuate itfelf deep among them. The tendon, inftead of inflaming and floughing out, became only foft, fpongy and

and dead; and never ſeparated unleſs it was cut out. We might ſyringe with all the cleaning and ſtimulating liquors we could think of; and dilate and make as many counter-openings in the foot as we pleaſed, and give wine, bark and opiates in any quantity; but where the matter had become black and gangrenous, and had inſinuated itſelf among the tendons in the ſole of the foot, we never got one of them to heal without amputation. Badly ulcerated toes, (which in other ſituations would have healed without difficulty,) were often obliged to be taken off, in order to prevent this danger. Latent and imperceptible ſcorbutic cacochymia may be thought to have been, and probably was in ſome degree at the bottom of ſuch a general tendency to acrimony and ill condition of our ulcers. Bark had but precarious and uncertain effects at beſt; and independent of this, we were often prevented from a free, or full exhibition of it, from bilious diatheſis, or a ſuſpicious condition of the abdominal viſcera,—an inflammatory or obſtructed ſtate of the liver or meſentery. Wine was allowed to the patients with as much liberality, (conſidering the price,) as could reaſonably be expected. Vegetable diet and fruits could

be

be procured but in ſparing proportion. The cocoa-tree liquor called *toddy*, we had, but it was of ſo fermentable a nature, as to become aceſcent in a ſhort time, and much of it produced diſorder and griping in the bowels *.

Our firſt application to all foul, ſanious and ſloughy ulcers, or where the edges were tumid, painful, and inflamed; and to all bruiſed and lacerated wounds; was fomentation with Decoct. Chamæmel. Flor. Sambuc. Summat. Abſynth. and poultices. Some people thought we were too liberal in the uſe of theſe; and continued them too long. It was an eaſy mode of dreſſing, and gave but little trouble, except to the aſſiſtants, or the patients themſelves. And no doubt it might often happen, from the great number of caſes poured in upon us at once after actions, or on the return of the fleet from a long cruize, and the want of ſufficient aſſiſtance at the hoſpital, that ſome irregularity in regard to dreſſings, might now and then take place. But it was oftener owing to the inclination

* See Appendix No. IV.

clination of the patients themſelves; they were generally fond of continuing poultices longer than was neceſſary;—a proof that they afforded eaſe at leaſt. Rice boiled to a conſiſtence to make it ſoft and ſmooth, or rice-flour with a little hog's-lard, made as good an emollient poultice as we could wiſh. To have made them of more fermentable materials, by mixing up a quantity of cocoa juice with the boiled poultice, might have anſwered well as an antiſeptic application, (if frequently enough renewed,) to our foul and putrid ſores. But this, ſo far as I know, was never tried. Indeed, the common rice-poultices, from the heat of the weather, were generally in a ſtate of fermentation before they were removed. Soft and oily poultices applied cold were abſolutely neceſſary for another condition of ulcers; where a tough adhering mucus, which could not be removed by wiping, or waſhing, was thrown out upon the ſurface of the ſore. This kind of diſcharge was only to be removed by poultices of this ſort; and then a pledget dipped in plain ſpirits, ſoon brought the ulcer to ſuch a ſtate, that no more of the coagulable lymph, than could be converted into proper pus was thrown out upon it.

Whenever

Whenever any portion of an ulcer got clean, and began to granulate, dry lint was there applied, while the poultice was continued over the whole; ſo long as the edges were inflamed, and the diſcharge from any part of it foul and ſanious; or till the whole ſurface became uniformly clean and healthy. But as the ſtate of our ſores was ſubject to frequent variations, either wholly or in part; ſo behoved to be our applications. It was no uncommon thing with us, to have a large ulcer dreſſed with different applications at the ſame time; perhaps a pledget of dry lint, or wetted with ſpirits, or aſtringent ſolution where it was clean, and a poultice over the whole, to digeſt and deterge inflamed ſloughy and gangrenous margins, or to diſſolve and clean away glutinous mucus.

In all caſes we made it a rule to renew our poultices three times at leaſt in the day, and to waſh with Decoct. Chamæmel. at every application; and if an ulcer, after being once clean, put on again a foul appearance, we always found it neceſſary to have recourſe to theſe anew for correcting the diſcharge.

Our general mode of dreſſing, for all clean and granulating ulcers, after inflammation of the edges

had

had fully ſubſided; was with ſlips of cerate plaſter, and country lint. This laſt was coarſe bleached cotton thread, without any dreſſing, made to lie ſtraight by combing it with a wide comb; and cut in lengths adapted to the ſize of the ſore. This made the moſt light and eaſy dreſſing I have ſeen, ſufficiently abſorbent; and it always came off with great eaſe. A long cerate ſtrap over each end, faſtened it down upon the ſkin, and kept the whole ſteady, till a compreſs and roller was applied. This was alſo of cotton cloth, and embraced the whole member. Upon no one thing does the healing of ulcers more depend, than upon the neat, eaſy and uniform application of this. A ſplit at one end, ſo as to give it two heads, makes it tie eaſily round the member, and prevents the uſe of pins, which are always troubleſome, and often wanting in an hoſpital; or they are getting wetted and ruſted, and unfit for uſe. Or perhaps they are left to the patient himſelf to put in; in the doing of which, he very often ſhifts and alters the tenſion of the whole bondage. *Baynton's ſtraps* may do very well, and be very uſeful in private practice, or in ſingle caſes; but they will never come into general uſe in large military hoſpitals, until

until these be much better provided with aſſiſtants than they are at preſent.

We had never any trouble with hard and callous edges; nor any need of cauſtic for their reduction; nor had we any occaſion for precipitate to produce incipient incarnation in the bottom of ſores. But we had much occaſion for the latter, and the milder eſcharotics and aſtringents, to reſtrain or deſtroy the growth of a ſoft, flabby, and ſpongy fleſh, which, whenever an ulcer got tolerably clean, was but too apt to ſpring up, and again become ſloughy and caſt off. So that cicatrization was often impeded by this looſe luxuriency, as much as by the laxity, want of tone, and due contraction of the neighbouring ſkin. Hence the great advantage derived from the uſe of aſtringents; and of all thoſe which we employed, none anſwered ſo well as blue vitriol, in ſolutions of different ſtrengths, adapted to what we thought the condition of the ſore. A quantity of dreſſing cotton, prepared by being wetted with this, and afterwards dried, was always kept in readineſs for this purpoſe; as well as a bottle or two of vitriol water, of different ſtrengths for waſhing, as the dreſſer judged preferable. Few ulcers were healed and

and ſkinned over without this application. But when the ſore was nearly cloſing, we behoved to uſe this but ſparingly, to avoid the danger of forming a ſcab upon it, inſtead of a ſound cicatrix; and when this was avoided, the cicatrizations procured by this means, continued as firm and ſteady, as where nothing of the kind was employed.

As the healing of the ſore goes on, it is always of conſequence to favour the contraction of the ſkin, by the application of compreſſes to the neighbouring parts, and to give a little more tightneſs to the bandage over theſe, with a view to diminiſh, as much as poſſible, the extent of cicatrix, which never has the firmneſs of real ſkin; nor is furniſhed with cellular membrane, to allow free motion to the parts below it: Though it ſometimes gets ſo hard and contracted, as to impede the circulation, and occaſion varicoſe and œdematous ſwellings. So that much of the future uſefulneſs of the member, wherever there has been a large ulcer, depends on the ſize and goodneſs of the cicatrix that has been formed. It is from this circumſtance, more than from the weakneſs of the new ſkin, that ulcers of any ſize on the legs, are attended with ſo much unſoundneſs and diſability of the member, and are ſo liable to open up again by any future violent exertions. If it has penetrated ſo deep as the muſcles, the granulations from them unite with the new formed-ſkin, without the intervention of cellular membrane ; ſo that the action of the muſcle has a continual tendency to break it up afreſh.

Sometimes our ulcers, with every thing looking well, and filling up with healthy granulations, with well-conditioned pus, would without any viſible cauſe become ſtationary ; and then we often found, that by varying the dreſſings, the healing would go on again very well ; very often by withdrawing the aſtringent ſolution, and applying poultices for a few days ; or by ſubſtituting ſpiritous applications, in place of the vitriolic water. And I often found, unmethodical as it may ſeem, that under the alternations of the laſt with poultices, a ſore would heal as well as with any ſort of dreſſing whatver ; the one ſo far counteracting the other, as to preſerve the proper tone in the veſſels neceſſary for conducting the healing proceſs. Whenever a clean and healthy ulcer becomes ſtationary, without a ſyſtematic affection, I am perſuaded

ſuaded it is from want of this neceſſary condition being maintained in its veſſels; and that we will often attain our purpoſe, by a little variation in our applications; and where we have no particular index to guide our choice, it will be found beſt to adopt for a time, ſuch as are of an oppoſite character to the laſt in uſe.

Notwithſtanding the general malignity, and ill-conditioned diſcharges from our hoſpital ulcers, whenever thoſe on the legs continued long, I obſerved, that they became a mere local diſeaſe at laſt; and a great deal of attention, pains, and judgment was requiſite, to vary and adapt the dreſſings and applications to every varying ſtate of ſuch ulcers, in order to maintain that tone and action of the veſſels, without which no good pus nor healing proceſs can be procured in any ſore. I am perſuaded, it is owing to want of attention to theſe circumſtances, and owing to the dreſſing of ſores being left almoſt entirely to the care of ſtudents, mates, and hired ſervants, that hoſpitals, military and municipal, have incurred the opprobrium they have long lain under, in regard to this part of practice.

Our amputations were all done on Mr Allanſon's plan. But where the weight of the patient's body was to reſt upon the end of his ſtump, we did not attempt to cover it wholly, ſo as to produce adheſion by the firſt intention; for this always produced much wrinkling of the ſkin, or inconvenient corners at each ſide of the limb. We found a better ſtump was formed upon the whole, if three-fourths or ſo of its circumference were healed up in this way; and we had the remaining cicatrix generally hollow, in place of being conical or puſhed out.

TETANUS.

In the year 1782, no caſes of this diſeaſe occurred at the hoſpital, either after amputation, or from any other cauſe. In the beginning of 1783, we had two patients ſeized with it. In one caſe, it ſucceeded the amputation of the leg; and the affection was but ſlight and eaſily removed by opiates. In the other, it aroſe from a gangrenous ulcer in the great toe. This toe was taken off as ſoon as the

the difeafe appeared. The patient had formerly been fubject to epileptic fits, which returned with the tetanus, and carried him off.

In the latter end of July, or beginning of Auguft 1783, on the return of the fleet to Madras Roads, after an action off Cuddalore, the hofpital lift was fwelled to the amount of 1800 patients, and the apartments were much crowded, notwithftanding of extenfive fick quarters added to the hofpital. Several of the fhips were but newly arrived from England, and the fleet had been out a long cruize. Many of the people were thus in a fickly ftate, or tainted with fcurvy. The land winds, which blow all along this part of the coaft, had not yet fubfided; but this is the ufual courfe in every feafon; and there was no other known circumftance, to which we could impute the furprifing prevalence and fatalaty of tetanus, which took place on this occafion.

Being employed, at this period, in the general management and regulation of the hofpital, and in dreffing bad wounds and amputated limbs, (which were very numerous,) without a particular charge, I had taken no exact account of the cafes, or of the numbers, that were cut off by it. Thcy were very numerous; 40 or 50, or more. It ſeemed to be all one, whether the tetanus aroſe from amputations, or from ſevere lacerated wounds, or from thoſe that were exceedingly ſlight, and in a clean and healthy ſtate; or whether ſuch wounds were in the fleſhy parts, or among thoſe that were tendinous; the diſeaſe almoſt uniformly proved fatal. None recovered who were attacked, except one; and in this one, the affection was ſlight, and confined to the muſcles of the lower jaw. It came on in this caſe from a bruiſe on the firſt joint of a finger. The finger was taken off, and the diſeaſe was ſoon removed. About this time alſo a ſimilar ſlight caſe came under my care in the Medea frigate, from a hurt or bruiſe, with fracture of the os naſi, and was removed by opium. It was quite another kind of diſeaſe in all the caſes at the hoſpital, except the one mentioned. It began with pain and ſtiffneſs in the muſcles of the lower jaw, but I never ſaw the jaw at any time ſo rigidly cloſed, as to prevent the introduction of liquids from the point of a ſpoon. The teeth could always be opened about a quarter of an inch or more, by a little forcing. A great degree of ſtiffneſs, rigidity and ſpaſm of the muſcles of the affected member

member ſoon ſucceeded with opiſthotonus and affection of the muſcles of the neck and back ſo that they lay rigidly ſtretched out at their full length. There was a peculiar ſhining watery look of the patient's eye, oppreſſion of the ſpirits, and ſighing, with a ſlight degree of fever, but no delirium or inſenſibility, In this way the ſufferers generally continued for 10 or 12 days, ſometimes longer, and gradually ſunk under the diſeaſe, without any change to the laſt. Some were not attacked till 14 days after the accident by which tetanus was brought on. Amputation was tried in ſeveral caſes without effect. The largeſt doſes of opium we could venture on both given internally, and applied to the ſores, and the ſtiff jaws; camphor, bliſters to the jaws and throat, warm and cold bathing and daſhing, wine, ſpirits, the volatile alkali, were all equally unavailing. In one caſe, full ſalivation was excited by mercury, with no better ſucceſs. Not one patient recovered, except in the ſlight caſe formerly mentioned; nor did any of our remedies produce the ſmalleſt mitigation, or ſeem to retard even the progreſs of the diſeaſe.

BURNS FROM EXPLOSION OF GUNPOWDER.

Burning from explofion of gunpowder was a frequent accident in feveral of our naval engagements; and when it went to any depth, was attended with terrible confequences. Whenever the burning was upon the head, neck or face, and the cutis vera was affected, the cafe was always attended with much inflammation and fwelling; and generally with fuch a degree of fever, as foon proved fatal. Indeed, but few recovered, where the burning was extenfive on the upper parts of the body. The pain and torture was fo great, and the patients fuffered fo much in dreffing, that it was with difficulty they could be got to admit any thing more than the application of oiled cloths. And if there was much inflammation and exfoliation of the cutis vera, this was followed by fuch an exceffive difcharge, as their conftitutions could not fupport. Very often the fever ran fo high, attended with delirium, hiccup and vomitings, as to cut them off in the firft week. We placed

placed our patients with burns in the cooleſt and beſt aired wards in the hoſpital, and it was neceſſary to give them laxatives frequently, as they were diſpoſed to be coſtive; and to allay the febrile heat and thirſt, by acids or tamarind water for common drink. But we did not purſue the antiphlogiſtic plan any further than this. On the contrary, we thought it neceſſary to ſupport the ſtrength by cordials, and ſtrengthening diet and drinks, as ſoon as any abatement of fever took place.

When the ſores began to digeſt, we found the oil cloths very inconvenient, by adding to the filth and uncleanlineſs; and that it anſwered much better, to waſh the ſores at each dreſſing with ſpirits and water, of ſuch ſtrength as could be borne without much ſmarting; and to dreſs with Ung. Alb. Camphorat., or, as long as the edges were ſwelled and inflamed, with poultices.

Of all the applications which have been employed in the recent ſtate of burns, I have never found any equal to the Carron oil, viz. equal parts of lime water and linſeed-oil; with an opiate in a doſe ſufficient to abate pain twice a day; with wine and nouriſhing diet after the fever has abated

Dry.

Dry powdered chalk recommended by ſome in the ulcerated ſtate of burns, is a coarſe and clumſy dreſſing indeed; and by its adheſion to the parts, and hardning with the matter, is very ill ſuited to the tender and irritable ſtate of ſuch ſores, but may be uſed in another way with great advantage. Apply all round the edges, pledgets dipped in linſeed-oil, or ſpread with any ſoft ointment. Powder the ſore all over fully, and to ſome thickneſs, with finely powdered chalk. Apply over this a piece of rag well wetted in linſeed-oil, ſo as to ſmear and ſoften the chalk. This converts it into a ſort of ſoft putty, which comes off perfectly eaſily, and keeps the ſore in a fine, clean and healing condition throughout the cure.

Deep and corroding ulcers were frequently occaſioned by theſe burns. In two caſes the amputation of the hand became neceſſary, on account of ſuch ulcers affecting the bones and tendons. In ſome caſes of this ſort, we found that a ſolution of corroſive ſublimate in water, employed as a waſh, did more ſervice than any thing we made uſe of: At leaſt three or four ſuch ulcers, that had reſiſted every other treatment, were healed up under its uſe. An impediment to the healing of ſome ulcers,

ulcers, originating from burns, and which had been obferved in other cafes, where ulcers were fituated over a joint, arofe from the action of the mufcles, on the fide oppofite to the fore; whereby the joint being kept bent, the new granulations were kept conftantly on the ftretch, and in a ftate of irritation. This was very obfervable in feveral cafes of ulcers over the joint of the great toe, and fingers, which were kept from healing, till this obftacle was removed by the application of a lined fplint along the oppofite fide.

FRACTURE OF THE CRANIUM, &c.

Nowhere fhould we fuppofe this to be a more frequent occurrence than on board fhips of war, and after naval actions, yet after three general engagements, in a fleet from 9 to 18 fail of the line, befides feveral actions with fingle fhips, two cafes of this kind only were met with at our hofpital.

The firft was a fracture over the fagittal future, of an irregular fhape; the bone cracked and feparated all round, of about the fize of a dollar, and

and without depreſſion. The crack was ſo open when he came to the hoſpital, as to ſhew very diſtinctly the pulſation of the brain, by the flux and receſſion of the matter reſting in it. No bad ſymptoms had ever occurred. The piece caſt off, and the opening was filled up with a fleſhy ſubſtance, in which new bone formed and united with the ſides in no long period.

The other was a ſimple fiſſure, of about an inch in length, in the occipital bone. No account being received with him, nor wound or hurt being known of, or appearing externally, he had been for ſome days placed in a fever ward, and treated as under fever, until his meſſmates gave information, that he had received a blow on the head in action. On ſhaving his head, a puffineſs and ſome diſcolouring of the teguments was obſerved on a particular ſpot; and on making an opening over this place, the fiſſure of the bone was diſcovered, with the edges diſcoloured, but not ſeparated or depreſſed. The ſtate of ſtupor in which the patient was, left no doubt of injury to the brain. The trephine was applied over the fiſſure, and an ounce and a half of purulent matter was diſcharged, but afforded

forded no relief, and he died in the courſe of a few days.

Little information can be derived from the recital of ſuch caſes, unleſs it be to remark the difference of iſſue in circumſtances, or from injuries nearly ſimilar; and that no prognoſis concerning this is to be drawn, from the extent of injury done to the bone itſelf; but from exiſting ſymptoms, as they may ariſe in every particular caſe. That a conſiderable piece of the bone of the cranium ſhould be fractured, and fully detached from the neighbouring parts, without being beat in, ſo as to compreſs the brain, may be difficult to conceive of. But many ſuch caſes are on record. It ſeems to be equally certain, that among ſavages at leaſt, many caſes of fracture of the cranium, attended with compreſſion, and with great and extenſive injury to the brain, are healed up without any aſſiſtance from art, or at leaſt only of the ſimpleſt kind. Thus ſays Lieutenant Watts in his account of Governor Philip's voyage: "At the "iſland of Huachuane, three of the natives came "on board, who had the os frontis fractured in "a terrible manner, but were perfectly recovered "from their wounds." Similar relations are given by by many other travellers and voyagers. Blows from ſtones or clubs, the common inſtruments of of warfare among ſavage nations; or falls from rocks or trees, muſt be the general means, by which ſuch wounds are inflicted, and muſt in many inſtances occaſion depreſſion, as well as fracture of the bone. This may be either with or without detachment of the depreſſed portion. How the ſyſtem is enabled to ſupport ſuch a lengthened injury to the brain, or in what way nature may operate to remove a depreſſed piece of bone, may be difficult to determine. A caſe I had occaſion to ſee, many years after the foregoing, ſhews to what extent the brain itſelf may ſometimes be injured, without producing any immediate effect upon the ſyſtem.

A boy about 14 years of age, running along the ſtreets at Dumfries, came with his full force againſt the foot of a lamplighter's ladder, carried horizontally; whereby a ſtrong iron pike, with which it was armed, was driven through the forepart of the os frontis into the brain; carrying all the broken pieces of bone along with it, and making an opening, within which the finger could be eaſily turned round. Yet he was neither ſtruck down, nor much ſtunned with the blow, and walked about

about after receiving it for half an hour, the wound diſcharging a good deal of blood, mixed with broken portions of the brain. He lived for 26 days after the accident ; nor until a few days before his death, that his left ſide became in ſome meaſure paralytic, did there appear much fever, or any alarming ſymptoms. There was a very great diſcharge of purulent-like matter, with broken portions of brain, and often in the latter period large quantities of clear lymph. After his death, the greateſt part of the right anterior, and much of the lateral lobe of the brain, was found ſuppurated and deſtroyed. The dura mater thickened, white, and detached from the bone, over the whole extent of the diſeaſed portion of the brain. And yet the pericranium, contrary to what might have been expected, cloſe to the edge of the original opening, which had been enlarged for the extraction of the broken bones, and another which had been made farther backwards, for the diſcharge of matter, kept perfectly ſound, and adhered to the cranium as completely as ever.

A method was adopted in this caſe, by the gentleman who had the charge of it, (Mr William Jardine, navy ſurgeon,) for enlarging the opening

ing made in the ſcull, in order to facilitate the extraction of the broken pieces, which perhaps is deſerving of being made known to the public. The object was to enter the trephine, without a centre pin. And it was ſuccefsfully effected, by the very ſimple contrivance of a circular frame of hard wood, (or the ſame may be made of ivory), of about half an inch in depth, and of ſuch a thickneſs, as to allow three well ſharpened ſteel points to be fixed in one of its edges, at equal diſtances from each other. The diameter of the circular was adapted to the trephine head, ſo as to allow it to move eaſily round within it, without ſhaking or vacillating. This was put down upon the bone round the opening, and kept ſteady by means of the ſteel points, while the ſaw placed within it, was entered with the utmoſt eaſe. The ſame inſtrument might be made of poliſhed metal entirely, and adapted to the trephine head, with perfect exactneſs, ſo as it may move within it without the leaſt ſhaking, and the bottom part might be ſcolopped out between the points, ſo as to ſhew the entry of the ſaw perfectly. It appeared to me that ſuch an inſtrument for entering the trephine, is preferable in all caſes, to that by means of the perforator

perforator and centre-pin; and for this reafon, that, whether the centre-hole be made with the perforator or centre-pin, this muft require much more preffure, and that directly downward, than that occafioned folely by the cutting of the faw. This may be of fome confequence, both to the patient and the operator in working on cracked or fufpected portions of bone. And befides, as the centre-pin muft always project fome way beyond the teeth of the faw, all danger of penetrating the bone with this, before the faw be fufficiently entered to take it out, is removed. This may be thought to be a very unlikely accident; but I have feen trepanned pieces of the fcull, with a hole fairly through their centre, in a furgeon's collection; and whoever will but take up half a dozen of fcull caps, and hold them up between him and the light, will be readily convinced of its poffibility.

The objection to this mode may be, that it will require a little more room and removal of teguments than in the ufual way. But very little harm, it is fuppofed, can ever arife from this. And let it be obſerved, that though the inſtrument may not, on trial, be found to anſwer ſo perfectly on an old dried cranium, it is quite different on a freſh and living bone.

APPEN

APPENDIX.

APPENDIX.—No. I.

Remarks on ſome Diſeaſes of Infants in Scotland.

THAT there is in the habit of infants a remarkable tendency to *bowel-diſorder*, and to *exceſſive fluxes*, we have the evidence of every day's experience to aſſure us.

Many circumſtances in their conſtitution combine to occaſion this. Among others is the irritation ariſing from *dentition*. This is generally ſpoken of, as if it were ſuppoſed there exiſted an eſtabliſhed ſympathy between the membrane of the alveoli, and the coats of the ſtomach and inteſtines, by which diſorder and looſeneſs might be produced, in conſequence of the affection of the gums. But there is no occaſion for this ſuppoſition; and the truth is, the diſorder ariſes wholly from an acrimony in the ſecretions from the mouth, the conſequence of inflammation induced on the parts, by the riſing of the teeth.

Another circumſtance is weaning; which is often followed by ſimilar complaints, called in Scotland the *weaning-braſh*, and is generally imputed to the change of diet, or to overloading the ſtomach with improper food.

I am however perſuaded, that both of theſe circumſtances are much oftener the remote and indirect cauſes, than the proximate and immediate; and that the complaint is much more frequently brought on, by what is very much overlooked; often enough attempted to be concealed from a miſtaken prejudice about the rearing of children, viz. from the application of cold. To the abſurd fancy of expoſing children at all ſeaſons to the open air, with a view to ſtrengthen the conſtitution, and make them weather-hardy, numberleſs lives are daily ſacrificed in this country. But when a faſhion has been once introduced, be it upon whatever irrational or inconſiſtent fancy it may, it has its run till a new one, perhaps the very reverſe, comes in and ſuperſedes it.

The

The idea of expofing infants, from a few weeks after birth, to all weathers that blow, except perhaps to a very ftorm, has been probably taken up from the cool regimen, and expofure to free and cool air, proper in fmall pox, and in the treatment of fever; and it proceeds upon the fuppofition, that an infant, born perhaps in a town in the beginning of winter, and to be brought up in all the delicacy of a city life, fhould be able to bear the application of as much cold, as the full grown fubject, or as perhaps its parents were accuftomed to bear under a very different fort of rearing in the country. All this, however, is contrary to nature, of which every mother may convince herfelf, in fpite of the fafhion, if fhe will condefcend to be inftructed by *inftinct*, which never errs. Every mother who has no other inftructor for her guide, endeavours to fofter and cherifh her young by heat. The modern fancy is to *cherifh* the young of the human fpecies, by the application of cold: And for fome time, or to the period of dentition, it goes on, without feeming to produce any bad effects. But as foon as this commences, the irritation arifing from it, induces a degree of febrile difpofition, whereby every other exciting cauſe is rendered active; and the ſame application of cold, which before would have produced but little or no effect, is now ſufficient to light up an actual fever. The child begins at the ſame time to cough, and has an unuſual flow of ſaliva, with an inflamed or ſore mouth and tongue. This continues for ſome days, but ends at laſt in ſome ſtomach-diſorder and a ſevere looſeneſs. All this appears inexplicable to the mothers and nurſes; for the child has not been more expoſed to cold than uſual. But they agree to call the cough a *teething cough*, and the bowel complaint a *teething looſeness*, laying their ſympathies as broad and wide as poſſible. The whole matter however is perfectly ſimple, and there is no need of ſympathies to explain it. The application of cold naturally enough excites coughing, and the acrimony induced on the diſcharge from the mouth, from teething, and from the effects of cold, together with the diſcharge from the mucous membrane of the lungs, all which, with them go down to the ſtomach, very readily diſturbs the functions of digeſtion, and produces gripes and looſeneſs.

This

This is the hiſtory and the cauſe of almoſt all the febrile diſorders of infants, and of what are called *teething fevers*, *teething coughs*, and *teething* and *weaning looſeneſſes*. The proximate cauſe of almoſt all of them is untimeous and undue expoſure to *cold*; and every mother may reſt aſſured, that no infant, or child, can be brought to bear the ſame degree of this, without danger of ſuffering by it, as the ſame child or infant will bear eaſily, when advanced to the adult ſtate: and that the cold-water waſhings, and the ſending infants out a-airing in winter weather, and all the other parts of the caſe-hardening proceſs, ſhould be delayed till the teething and weaning be over; or till the child be able of itſelf to tell how ſuch things agree with it, and when it ſuffers by them.

The treatment of *coughs* and of *catarrhal affections* in infants and children, may be ſafely enough truſted to a few vomits of ipecacuan wine, repeated at ſhort intervals. The ſyrups and pectorals that are often ſought for ſeldom do any good, and are ready to add to the ſtomach-diſorder and indigeſtion. Equal parts of thin mucilage of gum-arabic and Syr. Scillit. A tea-ſpoonful once or twice a-day maybe uſeful at times as a pectoral,

or

or a tea-ſpoonful or two of Syr. Althœæ, with from 10 to 20 drops of Tinct. Hyoſcyami in each doſe, will often anſwer better. But opiates in any form are to be uſed with caution in the beginning of the complaint, or while the ſtools are diſordered, and of an unnatural appearance. The practitioner has but little to do with the cough; but he ought to be aware of what in all probability is to follow from acrid ſecretions; and where the emetics do not open the bowels fully, they ought to be followed with two or three purges; ſuch as 3 or 4 grains of rhubarb, and double the quantity of calcined magneſia, for a child of one year old; or, what will be eaſier given, 1½ grain of calomel, well rubbed up with 3 or 4 grains of lump-ſugar; or Tinct. Jalap., and Syr. Sacch. of each a drachm and a half; and ſo in proportion for thoſe above it; but leſs need hardly be given for any age below. When, from theſe precautions being neglected, or from whatever cauſe it may ariſe, the looſeneſs becomes exceſſive, and the child begins to fall into the condition mentioned *ſuprà*, page 83, any further proſecution of evacuants would be attended with bad effects: and along with the other meaſures there

there mentioned, the following mixture may be ufed with good effect:

> ℞ Potio. Cretac.
> Tinct. Catechu,
> Tinct. Croci,
> Syr. Sacch.—utriufque, ʒij.
> Tinct. Opii gutt. xx.

A tea-fpoonful, or more, for a child of one year old, two or three times a-day.

Ten drops of Aq. Carbon. Ammon. to be added to this mixture, wherever the matters ejected from the ftomach, or paffed downwards, have an acid fmell. This is fo frequently the cafe in the complaints we are mentioning, that it may be in general added with advantage. Where vomitings take place at the fame time, add to it the Aq. Ammon. with Spirit. Nucis Mofchat. ʒi; to be given in the fame dofe, immediately after every fit of retching.

APPEN-

APPENDIX.—No. II.

On the Diſeaſe called Cholic.

A place is given to the diſeaſe called *Cholic* in all the Noſological Syſtems, and ſome of them diſtinguiſh it into ſpecies and varieties. A late eminent writer places it under the head of *Spaſmodic Affections* in the natural functions; conſiders it as of the ſame nature with *Ileus*; and ſo far from entering into theſe diſtinctions, he ſays: "It "has the ſame proximate cauſe, and is attend-"ed with the ſame ſymptoms as ileus, only in an "inferior degree; that the proximate cauſe is a "ſpaſmodic contraction of ſome part of the in-"teſtinal canal, and that he is well perſuaded that "this is the ſame in all the ſpecies that have been "taken notice of, and that conſequently the indi-"cation of cure is the ſame in all of them, name-"ly, to remove the ſpaſmodic contraction men-"tioned *."

In

* Cullen's "Firſt Lines."

In looking over some Notes, taken at Dumfries so far back as the year 1786, I find that cases had been met with, which, from the way in which the notes have been put down, had perhaps been taken up in this view. They are to the following purpose. That through the winter of that year, there had occurred an unusual number of cases of enteritis or ileus, several of them ending fatally, &c. That during the succeeding spring months, seven or eight cases of *spasmodic cholic* were also met with, of which the following account is given: "That the greatest number were in female patients, all of them about or above the age of "forty; but whether connected with any disorder or irregularity in the menstrual discharge, "is not mentioned; that the pain affected chiefly the region of the stomach, which was sore or "tender to the touch, but without swelling or inflation;—that retching and vomiting took place "in all of them soon after the first attack;—and "that the complaint was accompanied with jactation, straining and twisting of the body, much "more than is commonly observed in persons labouring under enteritis: but that the belly was "in general open, or easily moved by purgatives, "and

" and none died of the complaint;—that bleed-" ing and opiates gave relief in every cafe;—that" laudanum, mixed with fome aromatic fpirit, and" rubbed on the pit of the ftomach, was frequent-" ly fuccefsful; but that more certain relief was" procured from adminiftering it by glyfter, and" that it was neceffary to ufe means to preferve an" open belly for fome time after recovery, in or-" der to prevent relapfes, which were ready to" happen if this was neglected." Nothing is faid about fpafmodic affection of the abdominal mufcles; and it is not now known why the name of *fpafmodic* had been adopted to diftinguifh it.

Since that period, however, I have met with fo many cafes of fimilar difeafe, clearly referable to acrimonious irritation, induced on the alimentary matters in the ftomach or inteftines, by excefs in the ufe of fpiritous liquors, or by the ufe of improper and indigeftible articles of food, and accompanied with fymptoms of imperfect or unhealthy digeftion; as gaftrodynia, anorexia, cardialgia, and habitual coftivenefs, as to induce a conviction, that though there may be cafes in which the difeafe depends on the fame proximate caufe with

with ileus, viz. ſpaſmodic contraction in ſome part of the inteſtines, according to Cullen; yet there are many others, to which we muſt aſſign a different origin, viz. the preſence of acrimony, ariſing from diſordered bile and indigeſta in the turns of the duodenum, and where the ſpaſmodic affection is merely ſymptomatic.

This will be confirmed by the hiſtory of four different caſes, that were lately met with in the courſe of the ſame week. The firſt was in a young woman, ſubject to a variety of ſtomach complaints, and habitual coſtiveneſs, but who was in good health at the time of the attack. This was inſtantaneous, attended with ſevere pain, retching, and vomiting of highly acid matters; ſpaſmodic contraction of the abdominal muſcles, weak faultering pulſe, with coldneſs of the extremities. She died within twenty-four hours from the firſt attack, without the bowels having been fully moved, to aſcertain the ſtate of their contents. The abdomen of this patient was opened after death in the Royal Infirmary. The ſecond was a married woman, liable to frequent attacks of the ſame complaint, and labouring at the time under a bowel-diſorder,

diſorder, attended with gripes and a feculent purging. This was ſuſpended for the time, but was renewed by the purgatives given her for removing the ſtomach-complaint, and continued for ſome days. The third was in the wife of a recruiting ſergeant, and was referred to no cauſe; but I ſuſpected intemperance or irregularity in her habits of life. The fourth was a male ſubject, and the diſeaſe was plainly brought on by a dinner of beef and greens, eaten the day before, not in the beſt ſtate of preparation. The three laſt recovered; but two of them, not without conſiderable danger. They were all treated in the way mentioned *ſuprà*, page 184, to which this refers: Two that were full and ſtrong, with blood-letting, but no inflammatory cruſt was exhibited by the blood of either.

A proper choice of purgatives, both as to form and ſubſtance, comes to be a material part of the treatment of ſuch a diſorder as this. The Pil. Aloet. *Ph. Edin.* two or three every two or three hours, until ten or twelve are taken, or till they purge freely a number of times, will often anſwer our purpoſe well. In ſeveral ſevere caſes, I have ſeen

ſeen the following prove very effectual, and reſt on the ſtomach eaſily:

> ℞ Pulv. Jalap. ʒij.
> Magneſ. uſt. ʒß.
> Sacch. Alb. ʒvj.
> Tere ſimul. opt. et adde
> Aq. Fontan. ℥iij.
> Aq. Menth. Pip.
> Tinct. Sennæ comp. utriuſque ℥ß. M.

Two table-ſpoonfuls of this to be taken, ſhaking the phial, every hour or two, according to the ſtate of the ſtomach, and urgency of the caſe, till it operates fully.

Jalap, without proper preparation and admixture, is but a nauſeous medicine. Much depends on rubbing it into a very fine powder, with hard lump-ſugar; and by means of this, almoſt all the medical powders may be reduced to any degree of fineneſs we wiſh to give them.

A variety of other purgatives, or of combinations and preparations of them, may be employed. Almoſt every perſon has his particular form and choice in reſpect of theſe; but in ſuch caſes as we have mentioned, we can hardly expect to ſucceed with any of them, unleſs by paſſing them through the ſtomach, while the ſyſtem is conſiderably under the influence of an opiate.

Purgatives have been divided into the *draſtic* or *heating*, and the *cooling* or *lenient*. I believe this diviſion to be quite fanciful; and that, independent of idioſyncraſies and peculiarities of ſtomach and habit, they are all very much alike; and that no purgative in a doſe that acts fully, will leave any heating or irritating effects behind it. With reſpect, indeed, to the facility of dozing, they are very different.

APPEN-

APPENDIX.—No. III.

Diſeaſes at the Naval Hoſpital of Madras.

The Naval Hoſpital at Madras, while I did duty in it, contained double the number of patients ſtated in the report of the Company's Hoſpital, p. 210; very often a great deal more.

Few venereals were ſent us from the ſhips, nor were there many in the fleet. The ſeamen had but little communication with the ſhore. Little or no prize-money was divided in the country; and the eaſy ladies at Madras do not often venture themſelves on board ſhips. Indeed, from the modes of life, none but the very outcaſts of outcaſts could ſubſiſt among Europeans in ſuch a character. At Madras, there were to be found females of the ſame deſcription, as in every long-ſhore city in every other part of the world; but it did not appear to me that venereal complaints were very common among them. Their attention to cleanlineſs,

lineſs, their frequent waſhings, and other modes of management with regard to certain parts of the ſyſtem, perhaps in ſome meaſure tends to prevent the frequency of this diſeaſe among them. But of this I am uncertain. The report from the Company's Hoſpital ſeems to import differently; and I ſpeak only from what I obſerved among the people with whom I was moſt converſant. Among ſome officers who lived on ſhore, I ſaw ſome of the moſt inveterate caſes of lues venerea, attended with vile leprous phagedenic and herpetic ſores and eruptions on the ſkin, and which were not cured without the moſt miſerable wreck of conſtitution I have any where witneſſed.

The great bulk of *our* hoſpital caſes conſiſted at all times of *ulcers*. Of the remainder, the proportion and kinds would agree very much with the report given at p. 210. No exact general liſts were, however, kept with relation to practice; and thoſe relating to contract, and the ſettlement of accounts with Government, could not be much depended on in this reſpect.

Of *Fevers*, properly *remittent*, that is, with a regular diurnal *remiſſion*, I obſerved none in India; and I do not know that fevers, obſerving

any

any other type, come properly under this defcription. In many of our tertian and quartan agues, the patients were not, in the intervals, entirely free from diforder ; fo that it might be difficult to diftinguifh them exactly as remittent or intermittent, and ftill more with regard to thofe obferving the quotidian form. In the inland part of the country, there may be more regularity. But at the hofpital, the type was very changeable in all of them, and they very readily took on the continued form.

APPEN-

APPENDIX.—No. IV.

On preserving Health in India, &c.

I am doubtful whether, in ſuch a country as India, where there are ſuch evident marks of a prevailing torpor and want of tone in the ſyſtem, the common practice of ſtopping a ſeaman's *grog*, whenever he gets a ſore or ulcer, be founded in a due conſideration of the circumſtances; and whether, in hoſpitals, when a full ſupply of wine cannot be had, ſubſtituting *punch* in place of it, might not, even in the caſe of wounds and ulcers, be, under circumſtances, attended with advantage. The inflammation which we found in moſt caſes in India attendant on ſuch complaints, was not of that kind to be injured by a moderate uſe of diluted ſpirits. Indeed, it ſeldom ran high enough; and more ſtimulus to the ſyſtem ſeemed in general to be the main thing wanting to the cure. The ſyſtem of a ſeaman, habituated to a daily proportion of ſpiritous

ritous drink, cannot fail to fuffer confiderably in its powers, if this be fuddenly withdrawn. The difcharge from a large ulcer occafions a confiderable wafte of the nutritious part of the blood ; to fupply which, will require a more ftimulating and nourifhing diet than the ordinary fare of an hofpital, and efpecially that the accuftomed ftimulus the patient has had in his drinks, fhould not be altogether withheld.

As being connected in fome meafure with this fubject, the few following obfervations may be of fome confequence towards preferving the health of Europeans in India. They may appear of little importance to thofe who are acquainted with the nature of the country, and the modes of living practifed there: But let it be remembered, that we are not writing for fuch.

By far the greateft number of perfons who go out for the firft time to India, are in the early ftage or vigour of life ; and if they preferve health on the paffage, arrive in it in high fpirits, and with the European tone and vigour of fyftem in fome meafure unbroken. The open fea-air, and the exercife which they have been accuftomed to take on the fhip's deck, has infured to them a keen appetite,

petite, and a healthy and vigorous digeſtion; and the European habit of uſing a great deal of animal food in the meals is by no means repreſſed by a ſea-voyage. But no perſon in India ever takes, or can take, ſufficient exerciſe, either within or without doors, to digeſt ſuch a diet. The modes and habitudes of life are in that country entirely different from the European; and this produces a conſiderable diminution of the digeſtive powers; but the acquired appetite remains for ſome time, and the uſual proportion of animal food is perhaps indulged in, till ſome ſtomach or bowel diſorder occurs to check it.

New comers ought to be aware of all this, and that they are now in a country where the digeſtive organs are peculiarly liable to diſeaſe, and they ought therefore to diminiſh conſiderably both the quantity and richneſs of their diet. They cannot too ſoon adopt the regimen of the Europeans who have reſided in the climate, and accuſtom themſelves to what are called the native diſhes, which conſiſt for the moſt part of boiled rice, and fruits, highly ſeaſoned with hot aromatics, along with meat ſtews, and ſauces, with but a ſmall proportion of ſolid animal matter.

Provided

Provided every degree of excefs, that approaches to intoxication, be avoided, a regulated ufe of wine and fpiritous liquor will be attended with far lefs injury to health than a full diet of animal food. But any degree of excefs in thefe, which goes the length of producing any diforder in the ftomach, or in the procefs of digeftion, will be attended with the fame bad effects; and if hard-drinkers be, in Europe, proverbially fubject to difeafes of the liver, how fhall they expect to efcape in a country where this is in a manner endemic? A little fhrub and water, or Madeira and water, between meals, is ufeful, and in fome meafure neceffary, to keep up the tone of the digeftive organs, and to fupply the wafte occafioned by an exceffive perfpiration. But the *fherbets*, compofed of acid and water, and perfumes, are mere *rot-gut* drinks, nor are the Englifh beverages at all worth the price that is paid for them. It is not by acids and coolers, that the feptic tendency of the climate is to be refifted, fo much as by hot and ftimulating aromatics, eaten along with the food, and a few glaffes of wine or of punch after it. The fuperabundance of vegetable acid in the ftomach and bowels, tends rather to injure the bufinefs of digef-tion, than to promote it.

Another way in which fome young men injure their health on their firft arrival in India, is from a kind of falfe bravado, and the exhibition of a generous contempt for what they reckon the luxurious and effeminate practices of the country. They have perhaps heard and read much of thefe before their embarkation; and this leads them to a general contempt of the country cuftoms and manners, as arifing entirely from thofe difpofitions. They will not fubmit to be deprived of the ufe of their limbs, and be carried about, laid out at their full length on a *palankeen*, like a fick perfon in a European litter. Perhaps they will not even carry an umbrella, to fcreen them from the rays of the fun, but will ramble about, and take their former exercife in the heat of the day, till fome climate ficknefs is brought on, and teaches them effectually to diftinguifh between what the inhabitants of the country have learned from experience, as the beft means of refifting its unhealthy tendency, and their own erroneous and rafh conjectures.

There is another cuftom, which tends greatly to confirm the opinion new comers generally enter-

tain

tain of the ſenſuality and effeminacy of the European reſidents,—the univerſal practice of going to ſleep on a couch an hour or two after dinner; but this, the neceſſity of avoiding perfect ennui, and being left alone, ſoon reconciles them to; and I do not know that any evil ariſes from it, provided two things be attended to, viz. to guard againſt a too full meal of animal food, and too much wine, and that this reſtriction be not made up by a proportional indulgence at ſupper. To this, there is the more temptation in India, that from ſupper being at a cooler hour, it is apt to become the convivial meeting, and the more ſocial meal. In fine, ſtrangers, arriving in India, if they regard the preſervation of health, cannot too ſoon adopt the modes of living followed by the experienced European reſidents there, in the management of the whole of what have been called the Non-naturals; and, as much as official coſtume will admit, the light and looſe mode of dreſſing adopted by the natives, will be found far preferable to the tight and heavy clothing of Europe.

FINIS.